BACK TO YOUR FUTURE SELF

EXPERT ADVICE TO KEEP YOU ACTIVE, MOBILE, AND FREE FROM PAINKILLERS

ESSENTIAL READING FOR AGES 40 +

DR. DAVID A. WILDERMAN, PT, DPT, MS

ISBN 13: 978-1985384880

ISBN 10: 1985384884

This book is not intended as a substitute for the advice of a physician or physical therapist. Readers who suspect they may have specific medical problems should consult a physician or physical therapist regarding any of the suggestions made in this book.

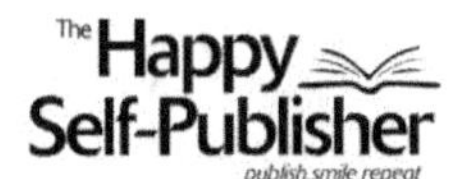

happyselfpublisher.com

TABLE OF CONTENTS

PREFACE

The World Health Organization (WHO) ranked the United States healthcare system as thirty-seventh in the world! What's remarkable about this is that Americans pay two to five times **more** for healthcare than people in most developed countries, yet we have one of the shortest life expectancies. Individuals can overcome these dismal statistics on life and health by investing the time, energy, and money that make health a high priority. Unfortunately, many individuals wait until they lose their health and then try and regain it. But that's very tough to do. Instead, you should do everything you can to stay vital and active by practicing good health habits in regard to exercise, nutrition, stress reduction, mental well-being, and rest and recovery.

We often focus on the term *life expectancy*, which some say is perhaps the most important measure of health. Ironically, it is one of the most misunderstood statistical figures. We hear the phrase and naturally assume it to be the marker of how long we can expect to live. Yes, it's true that today in the US, the overall life expectancy is 78.8 years: 76.3 years for the average American male and 81.2 years for the average American female.

The most naïve mistake a person can make is to assume that life expectancy is the age at which they will most likely die, but this would be incorrect. One definition of life expectancy is the age at which half the people born in the same year will have died. Life expectancy says nothing about how long an individual person will live. They could be in the 50% who die before life expectancy is reached, or the 50% who live longer.

The principal reason for our increased life expectancy is very simple: we don't die young. There are a lot more people living into old age because a lot more of them do not die in the first few years of life from what used to be killer diseases such as measles and whooping cough. In part, this is because of mass vaccination, but increased standards of public sanitation, better nutrition, and better housing have also played major roles. Keep in mind that in our country's infancy, 50% of children died before they were 5 years old.

Will our healthcare system be able to meet the demands of an aging population? According to the Global Health and Aging report presented by the World Health Organization (WHO), the number of people age 65 or older is projected to grow from an estimated 524 million in 2010 to nearly 1.5 billion in 2050. In addition, by 2050, the number of people 65 years or older is expected to significantly outnumber children younger than 5 years of age.

The WHO attributes the elderly population's rapid increase to a change in the leading cause of death—from infections to chronic noncommunicable diseases—which increases life expectancy. These chronic conditions may include high blood pressure (hypertension), high cholesterol, diabetes, arthritis, cancer, heart disease, congestive heart failure, and dementia. Heart disease, stroke, and cancer have had the greatest impact on the aging population. In addition, the incidents of obesity and falls are increasing.

This leads to the following question: what are the implications of the aging population on healthcare? According to the Office of Disease Prevention and Health Promotion, the first baby boomers (those born between 1946 and 1964) turned 65 in 2011. By 2030, it is projected that more than 60% of this generation will be managing more than one chronic condition. Managing these chronic conditions will increase the financial demands on our healthcare system. The cost increases with the number of chronic conditions being treated, taking into account that twice as many baby boomers are expected to require hospital admissions and physician visits by 2030.

According to the WHO report, some believe that as life expectancy increases, the prevalence of disability will decrease, because our progress in medicine will slow progression from chronic diseases to disabilities. As a result, there will be a decrease in severe disabilities, but increases in milder chronic diseases. Other researchers, however, believe that as life expectancy increases, the prevalence of disabilities will increase as well.

Certain health conditions are expected to be a challenge to our healthcare system with the increasing aging population. These conditions include cancer, dementia, increase in the number of falls, obesity, and diabetes.

Cancer

Due to the increasing aging population, the number of cancer cases is expected to increase to 17 million by 2020 and 27 million by 2030.

Dementia

The burden of dementia is expected to increase with the increasing aging population as well. Alzheimer's Disease International projects there will be 115 million individuals in the world living with Alzheimer's disease or dementia by 2050.

Increase in falls

With falls being one of the most common causes of injury in the older population, this is expected to be a challenge to our healthcare system. This is attributed to the fact that baby boomers are living longer, are remaining active, and are possibly on medications that could lead to falls. According to a report released by the American Hospital Association (AHA), more than 1/3 of adults 65 or older fall each year. Of those who fall, 20–30% suffer moderate to severe injuries (such as hip fractures) that decrease mobility and independence. Almost 350,000 hip fractures occurred in 2000, a figure that is expected to double by the year 2050.

Obesity

The number of people considered obese will continue to increase and have a negative impact on our healthcare system. Not only is obesity a risk factor for many health conditions, it is also very costly— obese individuals cost the Medicare program approximately 34% more compared to individuals of normal weight.

Diabetes

According to another report released by the AHA, the number of Americans with diabetes is expected to rise from 30 million today to 46 million by 2030, when 1 of every 4 baby boomers (14 million), will be living with this chronic disease.

What are some of the expected challenges we may face to our healthcare system? Here are some suggested by the AHA:

- Resource needs will continue to increase across all healthcare settings.
- The incidence of obesity will continue to increase.
- A shortage of healthcare professionals is expected.

- The diversity of caregivers will lag behind the growing diversity of patients.
- Care will be focused on a single disease versus addressing comorbidity.
- The sustainability and structure of federal programs in relation to the increasing aging population are concerns. As older people stop working and their healthcare needs increase, our government could be overwhelmed by unprecedented costs. Medicare coverage, which can be tapped into at age 65, could be pushed to its breaking point.
- Changes in family structure may lead to fewer family caregivers.
- Increasing need for long-term care—the number of sick and frail elderly needing affordable nursing homes or assisted living facilities will likely increase.

What is the impact of a growing elderly population?

There are great upsides to an aging population, like having more children who will know their grandparents and even great-grandparents. Healthy elderly citizens can share their wealth of knowledge with younger generations and can continue to make valuable contributions to society.

But over the next few decades, the aging population will face many changes and challenges. The majority of elderly Americans live at home, often with family, friends, and/or professional home-care services to assist them as their functional abilities decline.

Over the past decade, assisted living facilities have proven to provide a desirable living environment for those who require assistance. In addition, nursing homes remain an option for those individuals who require more intensive assistance, especially with basic activities of daily living. As our population ages and faces functional declines, older individuals may choose, or be forced, to relocate. Thus, elders may select living environments that optimize their health, safety, and functioning.

In summary, *longevity* is one of the greatest achievements of the twenty-first century. Maybe instead of saying life expectancy, I should really say *healthy* life expectancy, meaning the number of years a person is expected to live in a healthy condition.

The success story of longer lives is a worthless prize if the quality of those lives is compromised because of poor health and a loss of autonomy. Improving quality of life and functional ability among older Americans must be geared toward helping them effectively manage chronic diseases and complex coexisting conditions. After all, it's not only the elderly who are affected. But they can also place significant burdens on their families.

The factors that affect the differences between life expectancy and healthy life expectancy are many, but *do* include how much you exercise, what you eat, and the amount of sleep you get, as well as the burden of stress in your lives (plus whatever your genes have brought with them). Sometimes it seems incredibly difficult to do all the right things every single day to maximize your health and well-being, but of course the cost of *not* looking after your body far outweighs the cost of putting in the effort now. What are *you* doing to get more years in your healthy life?

Introduction

In the United States alone in 2017 there were over 140 million individuals with a musculoskeletal diagnosis, meaning conditions that affected your muscles, joints, and bones. In that same time period there were over 265 million prescriptions written for pain medication. Were you aware that physical therapists are the musculoskeletal experts?

Unfortunately, the most common treatments include pain medication, injections, and even surgery. And in the case where someone goes to physical therapy, all too often they are treated at a traditional "mill-type," cookie-cutter practice. This type of clinic deals in volume, so virtually every person with neck pain or back pain (or insert *any* area of pain here) will receive the exact same treatment due to lack of available time that the physical therapist has to spend with each individual client. There **must** be a better way! And I'm here to tell you that there **is**!

All previous treatments focused on the *symptom*—the goal was to make you more comfortable. The problem is that these treatments do not provide a permanent solution, and they require you to treat the symptoms on an ongoing basis—sometimes forever!

The *better* way to address any discomfort associated with movement is to see a movement expert—a physical therapist! But beware—not all physical therapy is equal. You need to find someone who has the expertise and skill to see your entire body as a whole, someone who can recognize that the *site* of your pain is not always the *source* of your pain. Someone who appreciates how the hips affect the spine, or how the feet affect the hips, or how the upper back affects the head, neck, and shoulders. You need an expert who is trained in *chain reaction biomechanics*.

Having been a movement specialist for over 30 years, I know what it takes to provide a comprehensive movement assessment that gets to the underlying root cause of symptoms. I then prescribe an individualized treatment plan based specifically on **your** goals and **your** lifestyle, not cookie-cutter exercises that are the same for every individual who suffers from the same problem.

You need a professional to *customize* your prescriptive movements. You also need a professional who is going to spend uninterrupted one-on-one time with you and not hand you off to an assistant or an aide. You need a professional who is also going to empower and educate you, so you can take back control of your life. If you're sick of treating only your symptoms, you want a solution, and you want to learn more about how to live your life pain-free, you will benefit from this life-changing information I have compiled in this book!

CHAPTER 1

How This Book Can Change Your Future

What keeps you up at night? Do you suffer from nagging aches and pains that don't seem to be improving? Do you fear that you or a loved one will be dependent on a caregiver in the future? Are you worried you will no longer be able to stay in your home for as long as you want? Do you worry about the rising costs of healthcare? Have you forgotten what it's like to be *normal*?

If you answered yes to any of these questions, there is definitely hope for you! I wrote this book to put your mind at ease. As a Doctor of Physical Therapy with more than 30 years of experience, I've encountered thousands of individuals who did not know the correct paths to take in their healthcare journeys, so they initially did nothing, and they needlessly suffered. And I thought to myself, *I can make a difference.* I already have with the clients I have treated over the years. But what if some of those individuals knew the secrets I am about to reveal in this book *before* they chose to see me professionally?

What you are going to find in this book are my top recommendations for making simple, healthy choices to live your *best* life. I'll address topics such as pain, exercise, nutrition, stress reduction, and mental well-being, as well as provide advice for rest and recovery. You'll get my best tips for how everyday people like yourself can understand how each of these topics are like spokes on a wheel, and how addressing each part will make the wheel turn effortlessly. These powerful suggestions, along with routine care from a skilled physical therapist, can get you back to living your *best* life and get back to being *normal* again!

If you require care, you should know that you have options. With the constantly changing face of healthcare, it is more important than ever to know where to turn for the best possible outcomes. An entire chapter has been devoted for you to explore your options in primary care and the differences in results when choosing a physical therapist. Finally, after I reveal how to find your best healthcare options, I'll show you how to stretch your healthcare dollar.

How much improvement could you make in your life by following the simple recommendations for overall optimal health I outline in the upcoming chapters? **You** have control to take an active role in living your *best* life, and I will show you how to get there.

Now I know some of you are struggling and confused and concerned. But with my lifelong passion for helping people just like you, I am confident you can get back to where you want to be. After all, none of us wants to be a burden to our children or any caretaker for that matter. None of us wants to spend our later years in a nursing home or rehabilitation facility. And we certainly don't want to be told that we can no longer stay in our own homes.

Wouldn't you rather be deciding where to go on vacation or which park to take your kids or grandkids to, or simply be able to take a walk with friends where you're not afraid of keeping up? Keep reading, and I am confident that you can make these small but life-altering changes!

CHAPTER 2

WHAT IS PAIN?

Pain. The mere mention of the word is enough to send shivers up and down your spine. Many of us deal with pain to some degree on a daily basis. It almost always has a negative connotation. Can it be that we simply don't understand what pain really is? Let me try and simplify the concept of pain to help you get a better understanding of what it is and why it should not be ignored.

We can't avoid it. At some time or another, most of us will experience pain of some sort that could potentially be debilitating. Some individuals tolerate pain much better than others. But why is this so? And where is the pain originating? Can it be that it is all in our heads?

What is Pain?

According to the International Association for the Study of Pain, pain is "an unpleasant sensory and emotional experience associated with actual or potential tissue damage or described in terms of such damage." So, based on this definition, pain can arise from *actual* injury to a tissue, such as muscle, tendon, or bone, or the *potential* for injury to a tissue. Regardless of whether the damage is actual or potential, one thing is certain—individuals will perceive pain as real!

How is Pain Understood?

Pain is one of the main symptoms causing an individual to seek medical help from a physical therapist or other healthcare professional. But our understanding of what pain is, why it occurs, and where it originates has changed significantly since around 2005. As short as five years prior it was thought that pain originated at the level of the tissues. (For example, if you hurt your elbow, pain signals originated directly from the elbow.)

It is now generally thought that pain is not perceived until the brain concludes there is a potential threat to those tissues. In other words, if you injure your elbow, then danger signals originate at the level of the elbow. Those pain signals are then relayed to the brain, and the brain determines whether it needs to respond by sending an output of pain. And this response is extremely individualized, meaning what causes one person's brain to respond may not cause another's to do so.

As a result of this shift in pain perception, the approach physical therapists use to determine care has changed as well. While many healthcare fields once focused on the treatment of individual tissues, many physical therapists are starting to adopt a bio-psycho-social model of pain treatment. This means that physical therapists no longer focus solely on the tissues of the body (bio), but now also account for psychological and social factors that can influence the amount of pain one experiences. This could include incorporating aspects of work or sport into your rehab program (assuming you injured yourself at work or while participating in a physical activity), as well as discussing any fears you may have regarding movement, and helping to give you the confidence to once again move safely.

How is Pain Described?

Everyone perceives pain differently. Physical therapists attempt to *quantify* the pain by having you assign a number to the intensity you are experiencing. "Rate your pain level on a scale of 0 to 10, with 0 being 'no pain' and 10 being 'call 911.'" Nevertheless, it is still subjective. What is labeled a 7 out of 10 by one person might be labeled a 3 by someone else. We often hear people say, "I have a high pain threshold," but because pain is subjective, science has not developed accurate ways to measure pain tolerance.

There are generally two ways a physical therapist categorizes pain: by time or by triggering mechanism.

Time-based classification

This is the most standard classification and takes into account *how long* someone has experienced their pain.

- Acute pain is pain experienced for less than three months. This type of pain is usually from a nociceptive trigger (see triggering mechanisms below), where you generally feel the discomfort locally at the injured tissue. This pain increases when the injured tissue is stressed or provoked and decreases when that trigger is removed. As an example, if you injured a tendon in your shoulder and you attempt to reach your injured arm over your head, you may experience pain due to compression, pinching, or stretching of that tendon during the overhead movement. When you bring your arm back down and tension is released, the pain generally lessens or temporarily disappears.

- Chronic pain is pain experienced for more than three months. This type of pain is often a result of a central sensitization mechanism (see triggering mechanisms below), which often ends in widespread, unpredictable pain. People who experience this type of pain may be hypersensitive to even the slightest triggers. Chronic pain is also very often related to psychological factors, and has been identified as a characteristic of the following conditions:
  - o chronic low-back pain
  - o chronic fatigue syndrome
  - o whiplash
  - o TMJ disorder (jaw pain)
  - o osteoarthritis
  - o rheumatoid arthritis
  - o fibromyalgia

The problem here is that these terms are used to categorize your pain, but they don't state the cause of your pain.

Triggering mechanism classification

This classification states what could be *causing* your pain, whether from a specific (localized) part of the body that is aggravated by certain movements (meaning the pain has a clear *mechanical* nature–called **nociceptive** triggers), pain arising due to damaged or diseased nerve tissue (called a **peripheral neuropathic** trigger), or pain that is usually *not* mechanical in nature and *unpredictable* in response to factors that normally increase or decrease pain (called a **central sensitization** trigger).

According to research, pain may also result in the following deficits:

- **Catastrophizing**: an exaggerated, negative orientation toward pain ("Due to this pain, I feel that I can't go on.")
- **Kinesiophobia**: a fear of moving or exercising ("I'm afraid to return to exercising.")
- **Fear avoidance**: intentionally not performing movements or activities due to a belief about the potential negative consequences those particular movements or activities would have ("My work might irritate my back.")
- **Inability to move** as freely as possible
- **Muscle weakness**
- **Difficulty performing** daily activities

How Can Physical Therapy Help?

First and foremost, your physical therapist should formulate a specific treatment plan based on your individual level of pain, symptoms, deficits, and goals. That being said, evidence suggests that simply understanding pain through educational means (such as reading this book) may result in decreased symptoms. *Know pain, know gain!*

Additionally, your physical therapy treatment plan should include the following:

- **Manual therapy:** This is specific hands-on techniques that may include procedures such as mobilization, manipulation, muscle-energy techniques, myofascial release, and other such approaches designed to increase motion and decrease pain.

- **Flexibility and strengthening exercises**: You may have heard the phrase "Move it or lose it!" Mobility and strengthening (in moderation) can significantly help you reduce your symptoms.

Take-Home Message

Pain is generally unavoidable; most of us will experience some form of debilitating discomfort at some point in our lives. (But good for you if you're not in this category!) You must ultimately realize that pain is your bodies' way of telling you there are problems. However, since you all have different perceptions of the intensity of pain, you sometimes minimize or avoid the warning signs, which, if unaddressed, can lead to dire consequences down the road. All the more reason to see a physical therapist before you reach the point where pain has affected and altered your lifestyle and has caused you to miss out on activities you love and enjoy.

Remember these important points:

- **Regular exercise is important**. Exercising on a routine basis has many health benefits, one being the improvement of the conditioning of the nervous system, which is responsible for sending pain messages.
- **Relaxation and imagery exercises can be helpful**. Oftentimes, pain can be triggered by noxious stimuli such as stress, uncomfortable situations, or loud noises, all leading to a heightened nervous system.
- **Bed rest is not always the best thing**. This is one area where our knowledge has drastically changed over the past twenty years. We now know that prolonged bed rest (more than two days) can

actually increase pain and lead to other medical complications.

- **Education is critical**. By better understanding what pain is and why it occurs, we can better guide our movements and activities.

Now you should have an understanding of what pain is and why it is so important not to ignore it. For the same reason you would not ignore the Check Engine light in your car, you should not minimize the type and severity of pain you may be experiencing.

In the next chapter, I'll show you how exercise is a key component in helping keep pain at bay, especially chronic pain, not only by helping to raise pain tolerance but by also helping to decrease pain perception.

CHAPTER 3

EXERCISE

There are many reasons we tend to slow down and become more sedentary with age. It may be due to health problems, weight or pain issues, or worries about falling. Maybe you think that exercising simply isn't for you. But as you grow older, an active lifestyle becomes more important than ever to your health. Moving can help boost your energy, maintain your independence, protect your heart, and manage symptoms of illness or pain as well as your weight. It's no secret that physical activity is one of the top contributors to longevity, adding years to your life—even if you don't start exercising until your senior years. In this chapter, I'll show you not only how you will look better when you exercise, but also how you'll feel sharper and more energetic, and experience a greater sense of wellness.

Benefits of Exercise

Physical activity means moving your body and using your muscles and energy more than you do when resting. Daily physical activity will benefit your physical, psychological, and social health. It is also one of the best ways that everyone—children, adults, and people with disabilities—can prevent or improve many chronic conditions such as heart disease, diabetes, depression, and some cancers. Other important benefits may include…

- Stronger bones and muscles
- Increased energy
- Lower blood pressure
- Improved mood and mental health
- Maintained healthy weight
- Improved sleep
- Improved concentration
- Improved memory
- Improved learning ability
- Decreased stress
- Reduced aging and menopause symptoms
- Improved ability to perform daily activities
- Diminished risk of accidental falls

There are some simple guidelines to help you determine how much physical activity you should be striving for. According to the Department of Health and Human Services' Physical Activity Guidelines, adults should do at least 150 minutes a week of moderate-intensity (30 minutes per day for 5 days) or 75 minutes a week of vigorous-intensity physical activity, or an equivalent combination of moderate- and vigorous-intensity aerobic activity. Children and adolescents should do 60 minutes or more of physical activity daily.

You may be wondering whether you should still be performing physical activity if you have a medical condition. The answer in most cases is yes, you should still do physical activity even if you have an existing chronic disease or condition. Make sure you check with your physical therapist or physician first to ensure you are healthy enough for exercise and find out which physical activities are safe for you. Remember that physical therapists are experts in physical activity for people of any age and condition, so you can count on them to help get you moving safely.

What about people with disabilities? Everyone can benefit and have fun from being physically active, including children and adults with disabilities. It is just as important for people with disabilities to do physical activity as it is for nondisabled individuals. Anyone with a disability, whether physical, mental, or developmental, should be physically active!

You may be wondering specifically how physical therapy can help. Physical therapists have extensive training and knowledge of physical activities and medical conditions, so they are truly the experts at creating safe and effective physical activity programs for individuals with virtually any medical conditions or physical limitations. Physical therapists also help healthy people learn physical activities they can do to prevent injuries and decrease the likelihood of chronic medical diseases.

Your physical therapist will most likely begin by testing your mobility and strength, reviewing your medical history, and discussing your health goals and favorite activities. As your fitness levels improve, your physical therapist will help you expand and advance your physical activities in a safe and fun way. The goal is to perform physical activities you enjoy so that you will look forward to doing them every day!

Have you ever been on a health and fitness rollercoaster? I'm sure many of you have—I know I'm no exception! You hear about a great new diet or fitness trend from a friend or see it on the internet. You do some minimal research, but really get convinced by the dramatic before-and-after photos, along with amazing testimonials. This prompts you to get new workout clothes, and maybe even persuades you to get rid of all the sugary foods in your kitchen in preparation for your new, healthy lifestyle. You just know this is the one that will work!

You're pumped! You feel great about this new healthy venture. You're happy…on a mission…committed. However, after several weeks of being "all in," the numbers on the scale have hardly moved. You stare at yourself in the mirror, but you're not really sure. *Do I look different?*

The novelty of this new routine has worn off. You're not seeing the dramatic changes you thought you would see from the before-and-after photos. You're finding it more difficult to get up early to get to the gym. The diet you were sticking to so diligently is losing its luster, and the foods you were able to limit early on in your "new you" lifestyle are now more tempting than ever. Are you forever doomed to failure? It doesn't have to be this way.

Why Diets and Training Programs Don't Always Work

The harsh reality is that every diet and training program requires work—hard work! It means working out when you don't always feel up to it. It means staying committed beyond the initial two- to four-week "honeymoon" period. It means staying motivated. But the fact is that many individuals are sucked in by marketing efforts. You are led to believe that these before-and-after photos are the norm, that you'll be buying in to a failproof plan to achieve your healthiest dreams, and that you'll see life-changing results in no time.

Imagine if you saw before-and-after photos of people after four months, and the photos looked identical. Or photos of individuals eating their favorite snack foods. Or photos of people struggling to make it through the simplest of workouts. Think you'd shell out big bucks for that dream lifestyle? Of course not! But what you end up buying in to is the ultimate outcome, the dream! That's what the marketers are hoping you'll do.

But when you get a few weeks or a month into this new, amazing lifestyle change and you're not seeing the results you thought you were buying in to, then you start having doubts—you start to lose your motivation, and you slowly revert to your old habits. "Maybe that wasn't for me," you say to yourself.

Why One Size Doesn't Fit All

You really have to go back to the basics here—everyone is different, and this is especially true with health and fitness. Your stomach handles food differently, your body reacts differently to certain types of training. While one person may love a particular type of workout, another may dread that same routine. Unfortunately, the advertisers leave out these nuances, leading you to believe that their product or trend is just what you're looking for, regardless of who you are or what you need.

So, what's the answer? What is the best workout routine on the market today? The answer is quite simple: the best diet and the best exercise program out there are the ones you can stick with! You must find a workout program you can do on a consistent basis. You have to get your body in the habit of moving daily, and you need to find a way of eating healthy that fits your daily lifestyle.

In order to get healthier, you need to be able to try different things and listen to your body so that you can make positive lifestyle changes that you can stick with for the long haul.

So, as you can see, there really is no such thing as "one size fits all" in the health and fitness world. There is only what will work for you as an individual. I'm by no means saying it'll be easy, because it won't! But the end result will be oh so worth it!

So how do you determine which workout program and which diet will really help you feel happy and healthy for the long haul? Start by asking yourself four simple questions to determine what is right for you.

1. **Is it something I enjoy?** Notice I didn't say "obsessed." But you do need to enjoy it enough to get past the resistance your brain will give you once the novelty of it wears off. And along those same lines, ask yourself the opposite question: "Is it something I dread doing?" If you answered yes, then this truly isn't the diet or workout program for you.

2. **Can I stick with it?** I get it—everyone has different schedules. Even though you may absolutely love what you're doing, the time commitment must be sustainable, otherwise you're going to burn out. An hour of cardio or 45 minutes of meal prep every day may not be right for you. So, start with a time commitment you know is manageable beyond a reasonable doubt. You can always add time down the road.

3. **Do I have like-minded people in my network to support me?** This doesn't necessarily mean

physical, in-person individuals, but you should have access to some type of community. Maybe you like to run. There are hundreds of running forums online where you can learn from and support other individuals who are pursuing a common goal. If you lack this type of community support, you may feel isolated, thus making it easier to quit. The same goes for dieting as well—you will benefit from a community of like-minded individuals who can provide recipes, tips, and support to keep you motivated.

4. **Is it working?** Check your progress after two months or so. Go back to a workout you performed in the beginning of your program. Can you complete it faster? Are you lifting heavier weights and performing more reps? You may also want to check physical markers such as blood pressure, body measurements (such as body fat), weight, and cholesterol.

Maybe you wanted to lose weight. Maybe you just wanted to tone up. And just maybe you wanted to be able to go for long runs. So, you went to the gym and spent an hour or more on the treadmill or the elliptical or the stepper. And you're proud of yourself because you've been sticking to your healthy meal plan.

But not all is right—the weight's just not dropping like you hoped it would, or you're having trouble completing your running because of nagging injuries. And you rack your brain, maybe blame your genetics for having slow metabolism. But truth be told, maybe you're missing something critical, like strength training.

Don't equate strength training with bodybuilding. Pretty much everybody could benefit from regular strength training, in terms of more energy, less stress, and better sleep. Would you like to know why? Here are 18 reasons you should be strength training:

1. **Stay injury-free.** Strength training is critical to preventing injury. Not only will you be strengthening muscles, but tendons and ligaments as well. (Tendons connect muscle to bone and allow for flexibility, while ligaments connect bone to bone and provide stability.) This means you will be less likely to sustain injuries from normal, everyday activities.

2. **Speed up your metabolism.** After you start strength training, you'll begin to notice an increase in your resting metabolic rate. Coupled with proper eating, routine strength training may help you lose weight more effectively than cardio alone.

3. **Improve flexibility.** Research studies indicate that moderate strength training helps to improve flexibility.

4. **Increase muscle.** Whether your goal is to lose weight or to get stronger, there is a lifting regimen that will deliver optimal results. This is much more critical as we get older, since strength training can help fight the natural decline in muscle and bone density that accompanies aging.

5. **Strength training can be performed anywhere.** This one should not come as a shock—you do not need a gym membership for strength training! There are numerous ways to start building strength at home that do not have to include weights or equipment. You can perform a very challenging program just from bodyweight exercises.

6. **Strengthen your bones.** If you thought drinking milk was the only way to get strong bones, think again! Strength training will help bones get stronger, which

can lessen your chances of fractures and, later in life, osteoporosis.

7. **Power up.** Do you have a desire to jump higher? How about to sprint faster? Strength training can work fast-twitch muscles, the muscle fibers used for generating power. You may just surprise yourself next time you play tennis, tee off in golf, or jump for a rebound in basketball.

8. **See results quickly.** You may be pleasantly surprised with how fast you can see results from strength training. Just starting out with two or three sessions per week can start yielding noticeable results in less than a month. What's that? You have no desire to bench-press 250 pounds? No problem. You can get an effective workout and build muscle lifting lighter weights (as long as you're still causing the muscle to fatigue).

9. **Get smarter in the process.** Well, what do you know? As it turns out, reading and studying are not the only ways to stimulate your brain! While any exercise can help keep your brain healthy, studies found that strength training resulted in better cognitive functioning in older adults.

10. **Improve self-esteem.** Strength training can certainly help to improve an individual's perceived body image. Think about tracking your progress so you can see your strength gains from week to week.

11. **Safeguard your heart health.** Eating heart-healthy foods isn't the only thing we can do for our hearts on the road to wellness. Strength training also has positive cardiovascular powers that can help to protect us from heart disease.

12. **Boost your spirits.** Not happy with things at home or at work? Research has shown that strength training can have psychological benefits, including feeling more positive in the home or in the workplace.

13. **Raise productivity levels.** Getting in a quick workout can help you stay focused throughout the workday. And if you can't get resistance training into your schedule, just taking a 30-minute walk during lunch can help to elevate your mood and decrease your stress levels.

14. **Conquer boredom.** Muscles need time to recover. Switching up your routine is a must, and your body will quickly learn to adapt to a new challenge. A few ideas would be to decrease your repetitions while increasing your weight (resistance), try a new exercise to make sure you're working in different planes of motion, or increase the intensity, such as you do with interval training.

15. **Prevent the blues.** It happens—sometimes we feel down. It's called life! Studies have shown that strength training can help keep anxiety at bay by causing the release of endorphins, our body's natural pick-me-up. There is also evidence that it helps to fight depression.

16. **Sleep better.** Many of you have heard suggestions for helping to fall asleep, like drinking warm milk, sipping herbal tea, or taking a hot shower. And while there have been numerous research studies linking better sleep to those who exercise regularly, some studies suggest that strength training in particular can lead to a better night's sleep.

17. **Improve your cardio strength.** Do you secretly hate running on a treadmill, or exercising on a stair

stepper or elliptical? Good news! A fast-paced strength-training workout (especially those aimed at building muscle endurance) can keep your heart rate elevated and may even count as cardio!

18. **Reduce your risk of cancer.** Research studies have indicated that strength training three times a week for six months led to a decrease in oxidative stress, which can lessen cancer risk.

I can't emphasize enough the importance of exercise. Exercise offers incredible benefits that can improve nearly every aspect of your health, such as:

- o Helping to build and maintain strong bones and muscles.
- o Helping to burn more calories per day to help maintain your muscle mass and weight loss.
- o Increasing your energy levels.
- o Providing antioxidant protection and promotion of blood flow, which can protect your skin and delay signs of aging.
- o Helping prevent chronic diseases.
- o Helping to improve brain function, protecting memory and thinking skills.
- o Helping with relaxation and sleep quality, improving your mood, and reducing feelings of anxiety and depression.

Inactivity can have dire consequences, and it's been said that *sitting is the new smoking*. Our bodies were designed to move. By combining all of these benefits with a sound nutritional regimen, which I'll cover in the next chapter, you'll really reap the rewards from a healthy lifestyle!

CHAPTER 4

NUTRITION

The previous chapter showed you why exercise is so important to your health. But exercise must go hand in hand with nutrition. I'm sure many of you are used to hearing the words *diet* and *exercise* used together. But diet here does not mean a fad diet. A fad diet is a diet that promises quick weight loss through what is usually an unhealthy and unbalanced diet. Examples are the South Beach Diet, Atkins Diet, and Mediterranean Diet, among many others. Fad diets rarely work, because they are so hard to maintain. Your body will naturally crave things you are intentionally leaving out, whether it's protein, fat, or carbs.

So instead of trying a fad diet, what you should really be aiming for is a balanced diet, or balanced nutrition. Why? Because every food group serves a purpose, and exercise makes these even more necessary by putting strain on the body and using up energy. Your daily food choices affect your health—how you feel today, tomorrow, and in the future.

In this chapter, I'll show you why good nutrition is an important part of leading a healthy lifestyle. Combined with physical activity, your diet can help you reach and maintain a healthy weight, reduce your risk of chronic disease (such as heart disease or cancer), and promote your overall health.

What is Good Nutrition?

If you asked 100 people what "good nutrition" or "healthy eating" means, you'd likely get 100 different answers. Some think good nutrition means eating fewer sugary desserts. Others think it means eating less meat or fewer carbs. Sure, all of these are simple and easy to remember. Yet all of them are incomplete. To begin to answer this, you must ask yourself this one question: "What do I hope to accomplish with my nutrition plan?"

All good nutrition programs must accomplish these three things simultaneously:

1. **Improve your body composition**. You want to lose fat and gain muscle. There are plenty of supplements, invasive and risky surgeries, and ridiculous crash diets that can improve the way you look temporarily, but they do so at the expense of your health and well-being.

2. **Improve your health**. Whether you have health issues that need to be resolved or you've got a clean bill of health, proper nutrition should improve your health profile and keep it tip-top for a long, long time. From reducing your blood lipids to increasing your insulin sensitivity, from decreasing diabetes risk to increasing good cholesterol, from reducing body fat percentage to increasing your lean body mass, a good nutrition program will not only help you look better but will also

improve your overall health and functioning well into old age.

3. **Improve your performance**. People choose many ways to improve performance, including performance-enhancing drugs, crash diets and diuretics (to make weight for competition), or loading up on pasta before a big race. Yet none of these are ideal for long-term achievement, and some of them compromise health and body composition. Thus, focusing solely on weight loss, health, or performance while ignoring the other goals can cause problems.

Keep these three things in mind when you think about nutrition. And keep this in mind as well—good nutrition is outcome-based. Theory is nice, but results are everything. Remain appropriately skeptical of all nutrition advice you hear until you've tested it on yourself and proven that it can improve your body composition, health, and performance.

Benefits of Eating Healthy

The practice of good nutrition has a lot more to do with action than it has to do with knowledge. You can know exactly what to eat to lose body fat, build muscle, lower your cholesterol, or control your blood sugars, but you'll still fall short of your goals if you don't actually eat those things.

It's very common to see people lose weight only to gain it back. They'll read popular diet books and never change their bodies, not even a little. People will hire professionals at gyms and health clubs but won't improve, and sometimes will get even worse.

So, what's the deal with all this failure? Is it just that the advice isn't very good? Sometimes, maybe. There's certainly plenty of bad advice out there. But 9 times out of 10, it's because people are just learning without actually doing. They're seeking knowledge but aren't applying it, and that's why they're failing. They are not doing what it takes to succeed, and then they give up, cursing the advice, their genetics, and the system.

Let's use the example of a baby. What happens when a baby first tries to walk? They fall down—a lot. If you were the child's parent, how many falls would it take before you would give up on your child? How many falls before you just assume that the child will never be able to walk?

I hope you wouldn't give up at all! You'd keep encouraging that baby until they walked, and you'd do whatever it took to ensure success. You wouldn't blame the carpet for being too bumpy, you wouldn't blame the baby for being too clumsy, and you wouldn't blame yourself for not having a degree in biomechanics. You'd just keep praising until your baby walked.

So why don't we do this with ourselves? Why don't we stick to our health and fitness goals until we succeed? Why don't we commit to doing whatever it takes to see change? Maybe because we've learned that we can take the easy way out. We have excuses. We blame our genetics, the system, a lack of knowledge, a lack of time. And these are all excuses for not sticking to our goals, for not believing in them enough to continue until we can "walk."

10 Simple Rules to Transform Your Body

The three most important principles of any diet are…

- When to eat
- What to eat
- How much to eat

When most people think of eating healthy or eating to lose weight, they usually think only about the third principle—how much to eat, or total calorie intake. But there's more to eating well, especially if optimal health, body composition, and improved performance are your goals. Don't get me wrong—total calorie intake is important, since it governs your total weight change. If you eat too much food for too long, with your intake outpacing your calorie expenditure, then you're going to gain weight. If you eat too little food for too long, and expend more calories than you take in, you're going to lose weight. It's pretty simple.

However, the quality of these gains and losses is what's most important. After all, you want to lose mostly fat, not lean mass. You want to gain mostly lean mass, not fat. It's the first two principles—what you eat (food selection) and when you eat it (food timing)—along with your exercise patterns that determine the quality of your weight gains and losses.

If you're paying attention to all three principles—how much you're eating, what you're eating, and when you're eating—you'll be in charge of your body, and your results will be light years ahead of those around you. Pay attention to these things and your health, body composition, and performance will fall right into line.

It will be easier to put these 3 principles into practice if you follow the **10 simple rules to transform your body**. These will provide a foundation that will allow you to control calorie intake, food selection, and food timing.

Rule #1: Eat every two to four hours.

Most Americans generally eat about three meals a day, with some sort of snacking between meals. This is not the best way to feed your body, especially if you're physically active. Research shows that eating every two to four hours is one of the most important ways to improve health and body composition.

Frequent eating (of well-chosen, properly sized meals) stimulates the metabolism, balances blood sugar, and helps maintain your lean mass while giving your body a reason to burn off extra fat.

So how many meals per day should you eat? Simple—just divide the time you're awake (say, 15 hours) by 3. So, if you're up for 15 hours a day, you should shoot for about 5 meals a day.

Should you eat before bed or before you exercise? Just keep the rule in mind and eat every two to four hours. If it's bedtime and it's time to eat, then eat! It doesn't matter what you've heard in the past!

Rule #2: Eat complete (whole), lean protein with every meal.

Complete, or whole, proteins are sources of protein that contain adequate proportions of all nine essential amino acids necessary for your dietary needs. Some experts will have you believe that protein is somehow harmful or unnecessary. It's hard to achieve the best health, the best body, and the best performance without adequate protein. Here's how to do it.

- Women should get 20–30 grams of protein per meal, the equivalent of about 1 palm-sized portion.
- Men should get 40–60 grams of protein per meal, the equivalent of about 2 palm-sized portions.

By following this advice, you'll not only ensure an adequate intake of protein, you'll also maximally stimulate your metabolism, improve your muscle mass and recovery, and reduce your body fat.

Examples of lean, complete protein sources include the following:

- Eggs: Egg whites, whole eggs

- Fish: Cod, orange roughy, salmon, tuna
- Lean meats: Bison, chicken, ground beef, turkey, venison
- Low-fat dairy: Cottage cheese, string cheese, yogurt
- Milk protein supplements: Casein, milk protein blends, whey
- Vegetarian choices: Soy burgers, tempeh, Tofu

Remember, protein is not just limited to breakfast, lunch, and dinner. Every meal or snack, every two to four hours, should contain complete, lean protein.

Rule #3: Eat vegetables with each meal.

Your mother was right! Vegetables (and fruit) supply important vitamins and minerals as well as helping to provide an alkaline load to the blood. Since both grains and proteins present acid loads to the blood, it's important to balance these acids with alkaline-rich vegetables and fruits. Too much acidity and not enough alkalinity means the loss of bone strength and muscle mass. So make sure you're keeping balanced!

A great way to ensure that you're getting enough vegetables is to eat two to three servings (a serving is about 1/2 a cup) with every meal. (So yes, you'll be eating vegetables every two to four hours.) Follow this rule and you'll be getting 10–15 servings of cancer-fighting, free-radical-destroying, acid-neutralizing, and micronutrient-rich power per day. This is one rule no one can argue with!

Rule #4: If fat loss is your goal, eat vegetables and fruits with every meal, and eat other carbs only after exercise.

To say it nicely, if you've got fat to lose, you've got to earn those higher-carb meals by exercising first! Want bread, pasta, rice, or sugary foods? Okay, but make sure you focus more on the whole-grain variety and save them until one or two hours after you exercise.

When it comes to body composition change, this carbohydrate timing strategy is the single most effective way to kick-start fat loss in people with stubborn and hard-to-lose body fat stores. It also minimizes fat gain in people building muscle.

Rule #5: Eat healthy fats daily.

About 30% of calories in your diet should come from fat. In practice, this can range between 20–40%.

Fat type is more important than total fat amount or fat percentage. Make sure your fat intake is balanced by aiming for 1/3 saturated, 1/3 monounsaturated, and 1/3 polyunsaturated fat. This will optimize health, body composition, and performance. Yes, we are taught to fear saturated fats. But when saturated fat intake is balanced with a healthy amount of monounsaturated and polyunsaturated fats, you don't have to be afraid of it.

Eating this way is easier than it looks. Just focus on adding the healthy monounsaturated fats (such as from avocados, peanut butter, or extra virgin olive oil) and polyunsaturated fat (such as Omega-3 fish oil supplements) into your diet of vegetables and fruits, lean proteins, and carbs when earned. Your dietary fat intake should balance itself right out.

Rule #6: Drink only beverages with zero calories.

Eliminate fruit juice, sodas, and other sugary beverages from your diet. While many people think fruit juices are a healthy alternative to soda, they have little nutritional value. And they're certainly no substitute for actual fruits and vegetables.

So, eat your vegetables and fruits, and drink water as your habitual beverage. Flavor enhancers, with no calories or sugar, are great for those of you who don't like to drink plain water. Green tea is another great choice, as is coffee (in moderation).

As for drinking water, strive for 8 cups (64 fluid ounces) per day if you're not exercising, and double that to 16 cups (128 fluid ounces) if you are exercising.

Rule #7: Eat whole foods instead of taking supplements whenever possible.

Sure, it's easier to grab an energy bar, a handful of mixed nuts, a granola bar, or a protein shake than it is to prepare a whole-food meal. However, it's best to get as many whole-food meals as possible. Eat bars and shakes only when you're crunched for time or during the exercise/post-exercise period when only liquid nutrition will do.

Don't rely on multivitamins—instead, eat a complete diet full of lean meats, vegetables, fruits, high-fiber nutrient-dense carbs (at the right times), and good fats. Of course, if you don't have whole-food meals prepared, you probably won't eat them, which leads us to the next rule.

Rule #8: Plan ahead for meals and prepare food in advance.

The hardest part about eating well isn't necessarily understanding which foods are good and which are bad. Nor is it understanding proteins, carbs, and fats, or when to eat certain foods. The hardest part is consistency. Sometimes good nutrition is less about what the food is and more about making sure the food is available when it's time to eat.

Therefore, you'll need to come up with food preparation strategies to ensure you consistently get the nutrition you need, when you need it. For example, I'll cook a bunch of meals on Sunday to have for the upcoming week. If that's not to your liking, you can get up 30 minutes earlier and prepare all of your meals for that day. A third option is to hire a food preparation service to do it for you. But it's critical that you have a plan. As the saying goes, "Failing to plan is planning to fail."

Rule #9: Eat a wide variety of good foods.

Many of us eat in a very habitual manner, ingesting similar breakfasts, lunches, and dinners every day. Boring, but easy.

It's important to include seasonal foods and healthy variety. Find healthy alternatives to the foods you usually eat. For example, use a variety of protein sources. Instead of the old standbys like chicken, beef, and eggs, try incorporating game meats like bison or venison. Instead of the same old fruit and vegetable sources like apples, oranges, bananas, carrots, and green peppers, try eating pineapple, mango, berries, apricots, spinach, kale, or cauliflower. And instead of the same old carbohydrate sources like bread, pasta, and rice, try quinoa, amaranth, or barley.

Rule #10: Plan to break the rules 10% of the time.

Look—nobody's perfect! It's okay every now and then to eat food that doesn't follow the rules above. So rather than expecting 100% adherence, aim for 90% compliance. That means you get to break the rules 10% of the time.

But be sure you're clear on what 10% really means. For example, if you're eating 5 times per day for 7 days of the week, that's 35 meals total. Since 10% of 35 is 3.5, you get to eat 3 or 4 "imperfect" meals per week.

What constitutes a 10% meal? A 10% meal is one that doesn't conform to the 10 rules. Did you miss your protein source with lunch? That's a 10% meal. Did you skip a meal? That's a 10% meal. Did you skip vegetables? That's a 10% meal. Down an entire pizza in one sitting? That's a 10% meal—or maybe 2! Get the point?

Now don't get too bogged down with counting 10% meals and worrying about exactly what's a 10% meal and what's not. You should look at these 10% meals as a source of pleasure, not stress! (Just don't pig out, though—eating meals that are three or four times the size of your normal meals is not the way to your goals, and you know that already!) Pick a Saturday night meal, or a Sunday brunch, and eat some foods you wouldn't normally eat. Then get back on track with your next meal.

How to Make Good Selections

Ah, the power of choice!

We always have a choice in anything we do, and that certainly goes for deciding what foods to buy at the grocery store. The ability to make the healthiest food choices when shopping (and eating out) is crucial to consuming a well-balanced diet. Eating well means eating a variety of nutrient-packed foods and beverages as recommended by the five food groups of MyPlate, (www.ChooseMyPlate.gov) and staying within your caloric needs. MyPlate is the current nutrition guide published by the USDA (United States Department of Agriculture). It consists of a food circle (actually, a pie chart) that depicts a place setting with a plate and glass divided into five food groups. It replaced the USDA's MyPyramid guide on June 2, 2011. MyPlate groups foods with similar nutritional value together. These groups are…

- Dairy (calcium-rich foods)
- Fruits
- Grains
- Protein (includes beans, meats, nuts, and soy)
- Vegetables

There are three basic keys for making your grocery shopping the most healthful.

1. Know your store.
2. Bring a list.
3. Review the facts.

Know your store. Grocery stores have thousands of products, with most food items grouped together to make your decision making easier. Many grocery stores have sections where foods similar to the food groups of MyPlate are shelved. Let's look at where you might find these groups in your local grocery store.

Fruits

Fruits are typically found in the produce aisle or freezer aisle, with canned goods, or at the salad bar. Choose a variety of fruits that are fresh, frozen, canned, and dried.

Vegetables

Veggies are typically found in the produce aisle, freezer section, with canned goods, in the pasta, beans, and rice aisle, or at the salad bar. As with fruits, try to choose a variety that includes fresh, frozen, and canned (especially dark green, red, and orange). Also opt for dry beans and peas.

Grains

Grains are typically found in the bread aisle, bakery, pasta and rice aisle, or cereal aisle. Whole grains account for at least half of your choices.

Dairy

Dairy products are typically found in the refrigerated aisle or dairy case. Choose nonfat and low-fat milk and yogurt, and fat-free cheeses.

Protein

Sources of protein are typically found in the meat and poultry case, deli, seafood counter, egg case, canned goods aisle, or salad bar. Choose lean meats, skinless poultry, fish, legumes (dried beans and peas), and nuts.

Don't forget to visit your local outdoor farmer's market during warmer months.

Bring a list…and stick to it! Healthy decisions start at home. Planning ahead can save you time and money, while also improving your health. Decide which foods you need in what quantity before you leave home! Base your list off of the MyPlate food groups to ensure a variety of healthy choices. Pre-planning meals will also save you time and help ensure you have the right items on your list. When you get really proficient at this, you will be able to create your list based on the layout of your grocery store. Make sure to get suggestions from other family members, especially children. Kids are more likely to try new foods when they help to pick them.

Review the facts. The nutrition facts, that is! The nutrition facts panel on the food label is your guide to making healthy choices. Reviewing the nutrition facts panel helps you compare foods before you buy.

So, what are your considerations when reading the nutrition facts panel? Make sure the following numbers are low:

- Cholesterol (less than 300mg)
- Saturated fats (less than 20mg)
- Sodium (less than 2400mg)
- Trans fats (try for 0)

Make sure you look for more of these:

- Calcium, Iron, Magnesium, and Potassium (check with your doctor)
- Fiber (at least 25mg)
- Vitamins A, C, and E (check with your doctor)

Also, whenever possible, use the % daily value (DV): 5% DV or less is low; 20% DV or more is high.

Note: This is based on a 2,000-calorie daily diet.

A Few More Tips for Healthier Grocery Shopping

Don't go hungry. Healthy eating starts with the groceries you have on hand. This is why shopping with a list is so important. When you grocery shop while you are hungry, you may be surprised at the number of impulse purchases in your cart.

Pick more produce. If you're like the majority of grocery shoppers, you will tend to undershop the produce department. You might toss a stalk of broccoli, a head of lettuce, and a bag of carrots into your cart and move on. Just remember— you're supposed to be eating 10 to 15 servings of vegetables a day. So as a rule, vegetables should take up at least 1/3—or even 1/2—of the real estate on your plate. So logically, vegetables (both fresh and frozen) should take up at least 1/3 of your grocery cart!

Stock up on canned foods. A lot of shoppers overlook the canned food aisle simply because they do not realize that canned fruits and vegetables can be just as nutritious as fresh and frozen, and canned foods are always available. Several research studies have found that meals prepared at home contain, on average, 200 calories less than meals prepared from restaurants—and they're lower in fat and sodium. Having a well-stocked pantry can lead to pounds lost and money saved!

Go plain. You will often find that the original versions (plain-flavor) of foods and beverages, such as cereals, yogurt, soy milk, and pasta sauces, are usually the most nutritious. This is most likely because, as brands extend product lines, they tend to move into more decadent offerings that cost more and have worse nutritional profiles.

Read the label. This is really just to hammer home the abovementioned key to use the facts! Bypass the front of the package and rely mainly on the nutrition facts panel and ingredients list. If you're looking to increase fiber or protein intake, or to lower fat/saturated fat intake, the nutrition panel can be a one-stop shop for all nutrients and can simplify the process of comparing products. Just check the serving size to ensure it's a reasonable portion for you. If not, you might have to double or triple the numbers.

Don't buy items at eye level. Name brands pay higher slotting fees to be placed on shelves or in displays at grocery stores at eye level, and those costs are typically passed on to consumers. Instead, look high and low on store shelves for the least expensive—and often the most nutritious—items.

Do one final check. Review your cart one last time before you get in the checkout line. Make sure your cart has 50% fruits and vegetables, 25% lean and plant proteins, and 25%

whole grains. Also confirm that you have enough healthy fats such as avocados, nuts, and seeds. Remember—you're only as healthy as your most recent trip to the grocery store!

Now you should have a better understanding of why good nutrition is so critical to a healthy lifestyle, and why nutrition and exercise not only complement each other but also depend on each other. Even if you eat a perfectly balanced diet, you need exercise to burn the calories. You also need exercise to strengthen your muscles. Your food gives you energy, and you need energy to exercise. Then after you exercise, you need food to restore your energy.

We can't overlook other important health factors of exercise and nutrition, such as stress reduction and mental well-being. Let's dive in!

CHAPTER 5

Stress Reduction and Mental Well-Being

In the previous two chapters, we looked at how exercise and nutrition go hand in hand for overall optimal health. But your body is not the only thing that benefits. Regular exercise and proper nutrition can have a profoundly positive impact on your mental health as well, especially in terms of depression and anxiety. These things also help to reduce stress, sharpen your memory and thinking, boost your self-esteem, give you more energy and a stronger resilience, and even help you sleep better. Read on to understand the psychological factors of a quality life and how to reap the mental health benefits of exercise and nutrition. It's easier than you think!

Managing health requires understanding the influence of psychological factors such as attitude, mood, and overall quality of life.

Attitudes are changeable. They can be formed from an individual's past and present. They can also influence a person's behavior and well-being. Some attitudes are deliberately formed (in other words, *explicit*), while others are unconscious or outside of awareness (that is, *implicit*).

Explicit and implicit attitudes both affect behavior, but in different ways. The kind of attitude we hold about a particular individual, event, or idea influences how we behave relative to it and, thus, how we experience stress in relation to it. Stress is highly correlated with both physical and mental health, so if we hold a certain attitude toward something that increases our stress level, our health may suffer as a result.

Moods also play an important role in both mental and physical health. Negative moods can influence people's behavior by determining how they interpret and translate the world around them. Interpreting an event in a negative way is a risk factor for a host of mental health problems including anxiety, depression, aggression, low self-esteem, and physiological stress, all of which negatively impact one's health and well-being. Positive moods, on the contrary, are thought to increase the likelihood of physical health and well-being by lowering these risk factors.

Optimism is a world view that helps us interpret situations and events as being generally optimal or favorable. Research shows that optimism directly correlates with physical health, including a lower likelihood of cardiovascular disease, stroke, depression, and cancer. It also directly correlates with mental health, as optimists are more hopeful, have increased senses of peace and well-being, and embrace change. In addition, optimists have been shown to live healthier lifestyles (for example, smoking less, being more physically active, eating healthier foods, and drinking less alcohol).

Pessimism, in contrast, is the belief that you have no control over the events in your life. Also referred to as learned helplessness, it is associated with anxiety and depression, both of which threaten your physical and mental well-being. It can also contribute to poor health when you neglect diet, exercise, and medical treatment, incorrectly believing that you have no power to change yourself.

The more individuals perceive events as uncontrollable, the more stress they experience, and the less hope they feel about making changes in their lives. Research has shown that people with a pessimistic outlook are more likely to suffer from depression and stress, to have weakened immune systems, and to be more vulnerable to minor ailments such as colds and fevers, as well as major illnesses such as heart attacks and cancer. They also recover less effectively from health problems.

Quality of life is now recognized as an extremely important healthcare topic. In general, quality of life is an individual's assessment of their general well-being (or lack thereof). This includes all emotional, social, and physical aspects of the person's life. In terms of healthcare, quality of life is an assessment of how the individual's well-being may affect, or be affected by, a disease, disorder, or disability. An individual's perceived quality of life is often influenced by their personal expectations, which can vary over time based on environmental influences.

How Your Mental Well-Being Affects Your Mobility and Physical Well-Being

You hear messages daily about the value of exercise and a healthy diet to improve or maintain your physical health. You accept this to be true, and at various times throughout your lives, you make conscious efforts to improve or maintain your physical health.

Mental health is also important to our well-being, but the reasons for this are often not as obvious. The World Health Organization (WHO) defines health as "a state of complete physical, mental, and social well-being and not merely the absence of infirmity." The perceived disconnect between mind and body creates the misconception that mental illness is not a physical disease. In reality, mental health has a direct impact on your physical health.

Most people have no idea how common mental illness is in the United States. Research states that one in five adults has a mental illness in any given year. Mental illness is much more than just being depressed. It covers a wide range of problems, spanning from ones that affect mood to those that affect thinking or behavior. Some examples include…

- Addictive behaviors
- Anxiety disorders
- Bipolar disorder
- Depression
- Eating disorders
- Schizophrenia

You may be asking yourself, "Exactly how does my mental health affect my physical health?" First off, poor mental health can affect your ability to make healthy decisions and fight off chronic diseases. Also, neglecting your mental health can lead to more serious health complications such as the following:

- Asthma
- Cardiovascular (heart) disease
- Gastrointestinal problems

- Hypertension (high blood pressure)
- Musculoskeletal problems
- Obesity
- Premature death
- Weakened immune system

Depression alone can cause chronic fatigue, insomnia, and increased sensitivity to aches and pains due to abnormal functioning of neurotransmitters in the brain. Add to this the issue that people with mental health conditions are less likely to receive the physical care they are entitled to. Mental health service users are statistically less likely to receive routine checks (such as blood pressure, weight, and cholesterol) that might detect symptoms of these health conditions earlier. They are also less likely to be offered help to give up smoking, reduce alcohol consumption, or improve their diet.

What are some things you can do to improve or maintain good mental health and physical health?

- Get regular exercise throughout the week.
- Eat a healthy, well-balanced diet.
- Get enough sleep so you feel refreshed when you wake.
- Spend time with family members and friends who care about you.
- Pay attention to how you are feeling and what your body might need.
- Make time for activities you enjoy, such as hobbies.
- Set goals that are realistic and achievable.
- Know that you are not alone, that there is someone who can support you even if it seems they are hard to find.

- Seek professional help for support if necessary.

As you can see, your body's physical health cannot be separated from your mental health. Each affects the other in complex ways. Symptoms of poor mental health can be disruptive to an individual's daily life and can limit potential and place stress on relationships. Paying attention to your mental health and making efforts to maintain and improve your mental health can not only benefit you psychologically and in your relationships with others, it can also support good physical health.

How to Get in the Right Frame of Mind

We have heard it from an early age—maintaining an active lifestyle should be one of our priorities in life. Only by taking care of ourselves do we stand a chance of being the kind of people we strive to be at home with our loved ones, on the job, and in our communities. And I'll be the first to admit that it's not easy!

Our jobs, in particular, can get in the way of working out, which kind of makes it paradoxical—the more challenging and demanding a job gets, we often struggle to find time to work out. Yet, we can't afford not to exercise because it is so important to our sustained success.

So, to try and get to the heart of this paradox, I compiled five tips for how to fit exercise into your daily routine, no matter how busy you are. Please note: Each tip is equally important. So, let's look at how you can stay fit despite a demanding job or life.

Cater to your own likes and dislikes.

You need to be realistic and know yourself. So maybe you hate to run…or lift weights…or do yoga. And that's okay! One person's yoga is another person's running or weight training or dance. You need self-discipline when it comes to exercising, so make it easier on yourself by choosing a form of exercise that fits your lifestyle, personality, and taste. Can't decide what it is that you like to do? Don't be afraid to experiment with different forms of exercise until you find what works best for you.

Work out efficiently.

Choose a workout form that you can do almost anywhere, whether you're on the road traveling or getting home late from the office. Ideally, it will be a form of exercise that doesn't require much preparation but accomplishes significant physical gains in a short period of time. (Sorry, golfers!) High-intensity interval training (HIIT), bodyweight exercises, and running are all great choices.

Make a schedule and commit to it.

How many times have you said (or heard someone else say), "I'm just swamped at work today. No way will I be able to make my [yoga, Pilates, spinning, swimming] class today."? That's just an excuse! What if you unexpectedly had to pick up your child or grandchild from school and had no backup plan? How would you deal with the situation? Would you cancel a scheduled meeting? Take work home with you? Do some hard prioritizing?

When you really need to, you'll get out of the office at the time that is necessary. Make a schedule, write it down (or add it to your online calendar), stick to it, and remind yourself that exercising is a priority worth keeping.

Track your activity levels.

There's an old saying that goes something like "If you don't measure it, it doesn't exist." Okay, maybe that's a slight exaggeration, but there really is some truth to this, especially when it comes to exercise. Make a note in your calendar every time you work out and add up your workout sessions at the end of each week, month, and year so you can monitor your progress and identify areas for improvement. Measuring your activity levels (and ideally keeping notes on your progress) can help you stay on track and realize when you're slipping before you've completely lost the habit.

Choose something over nothing.

You don't need an hour—or even 30 minutes—to get a complete, effective workout. And any exercises are better than no exercises. Heck, even 10 minutes can make a difference! You can always find a few free minutes in your day. That just might mean adjusting some of your tasks and priorities. With an effective program that is performed frequently enough, short and fast workouts can do wonders for both body and mind. So, squeeze in fitness wherever you are and no matter how much time you have—bodyweight exercises, fitness or exercise apps with pre-programmed short workouts, or you can even do some exercises right at your desk!

The bottom line? We're all busy, but even the busiest of us must keep in shape and prioritize our health. So, commit to making exercise a priority in your life, and never settle for less than feeling fit and strong.

Many times, we think some tasks must be sacrificed—and often that sacrifice turns out to be exercise. But what if we didn't have to sacrifice anything? What if we really could fit it all into our daily routines?

The hardest part of doing anything is often just showing up. And yes, when it comes to exercise, it's easy to think up dozens of excuses to put your workout time on the back burner. But a very simple way to stay committed and turn exercise into a no-brainer is to schedule it! It can take as little as 18 days to form a new habit (although on average, it takes 66 days for most of us). So, penciling in workout sessions ahead of time—just as you would for an important meeting or a friend's birthday—is one way to get yourself in gear for the long haul.

Here are my top seven ways to generate an action plan for creating and sticking to a successful workout routine.

1. **There's a calendar app for that.** Thank goodness for technology! Whether it's creating a Google calendar or setting a reminder on your phone, schedule your workouts on your smart device to keep in check anywhere you go.

2. **Use time wisely.** When your goal is to make your exercise routine consistent, even a shorter-than-normal workout session is better than none. So, if you're short on time, go for quality and not quantity! High-intensity interval training (HIIT) is great for a short exercise routine that gets your heart rate pumping without fighting the clock.

3. **Be accountable.** Meet a friend at the gym or to go for a run, book a personal training session, or sign up for dance lessons. It's a lot tougher to ditch workout plans if someone is waiting for you. And as an added bonus, quality time with friends makes the time go by even faster!

4. **Be realistic.** Are you one to hit the snooze button five times each morning? Then an early-morning fitness routine is probably not going to last too long! Making sure you exercise at a convenient time will help you stick to your routine better.

5. **Add some variety.** Schedules are great when you're first starting your exercise routine, but like anything else, even the most exciting workouts can start to get boring, thus making them easier to skip after a while. Whatever your goals or interests, try designating different days for different workouts—like a cardio class on Monday,

strength training on Wednesday, and yoga or Pilates on Friday.

6. **Stay flexible.** Even the best-laid plans can go awry. Family obligations, work deadlines, or travel plans can all get in the way of your scheduled workouts. Do not beat yourself up if you miss a workout! Instead, focus on eating well, stretching, or making whatever healthier choices are possible until you can get back into the groove and jump into your next scheduled workout as soon as possible.

7. **Have fun.** Yes, seriously! The more enjoyable the workout, the more likely you are to stick with it. Don't like riding bikes? Then don't waste your time in a spinning class! A word of caution, though—give activities a fair chance before you write them off for good. Although the first 5 to 10 minutes of a workout might be unpleasant, the exercise high you get at the end just might make up for it (and thus, keep you going back for more)!

So yes, working out can be hard. But making time in your schedule for some fun, effective, and tailor-made "you" time can make exercising regularly a true reward, and not a chore.

Support Systems/Circle of Friends/Family

Stress is a normal and unavoidable part of life, but excessive stress can affect your emotional and physical well-being. Emotional support is an important factor for being able to deal with life's difficulties. Loneliness has been associated with a wide variety of health problems including high blood pressure, cardiovascular disease, diminished immunity, and cognitive decline. In fact, low levels of social support have even been linked to increased risk of death from cardiovascular disease, infectious diseases, and cancer. The good news is that there are ways to seek out such support, and to nurture your supportive relationships.

As important as social support is, some Americans don't feel they have access to this valuable resource. When asked whether there was someone they could ask for emotional support, such as talking about problems or getting help in making difficult decisions, 70% said yes. However, more than half (55%) also said they could use a little more emotional support.

In fact, according to experts, almost every one of us benefits from social and emotional support. And though it may seem counterintuitive, having strong social support can actually make you better able to cope with problems on your own by improving your self-esteem. And you don't need a huge network of family and friends to benefit. Many people find camaraderie among just a handful of people—coworkers, neighbors, or friends from their church or religious institution, for example.

So how exactly do you go about growing your support network? Here are some suggestions.

Be proactive. People often expect others to reach out to them and then feel rejected when they don't go out of their way to do so. Make time for family and friends. Reach out to lend a hand or just to say hello. If you're there for others, there's a greater chance they'll be there for you as well. In fact, when it comes to longevity, providing social support to family and friends may be even more important than receiving it.

Follow your interests. Do you like to take walks, play tennis or golf, or read? Then try connecting with individuals who have the same interests as you. Join a club, sign up for a class, or take on a volunteer position. Just be realistic and know that it will take time for relationships to develop.

Cast a wide net. When it comes to social support, one size does not fit all. You may not have one person you can confide in about everything, and that's all right. Look to different relationships for different kinds of support. Just make sure you seek out those people you can trust and rely on, to avoid disappointing, negative interactions that can make you feel worse.

Take advantage of technology. Many of us prefer to sit down with a family member or friend face-to-face, but it is not always possible. These days there is no shortage of technology to help you stay connected with loved ones. Send a text or email or do a video chat. Just don't rely solely on digital connections, as face-to-face interactions are most beneficial.

Seek out peer support. If you happen to be dealing with a particularly stressful situation, such as caring for an ailing family member or dealing with a chronic illness, you may not find the support you need from your current network. Consider joining a support group to meet others who are dealing with similar challenges.

Don't be afraid to ask for help. If you don't have a strong support network and are not sure where to begin, there are plenty of resources you can turn to. First off, your physical therapist or physician can provide you with some helpful suggestions. Also, senior and community centers, local libraries, places of worship, and local branches of national organizations such as the YMCA or YWCA can help you identify services, support groups, and other programs in your community.

How Pets Help to Reduce Stress

When thinking of ways to reduce stress in life, usually techniques like meditation, yoga, and journaling come to mind. These are great techniques, to be sure. But getting a new best friend can also have many stress-relieving and health benefits. While human friends provide great social support and come with some fabulous benefits, let's look at the benefits of furry friends: cats and dogs!

Unless someone really dislikes or is allergic to animals, or is too busy to care for one properly, pets can provide excellent social support, stress relief, and other health benefits—perhaps more than people do! The following are additional health benefits of pets.

Pets can improve your mood.

For those who love animals, it's virtually impossible to stay in a bad mood when loving puppy eyes meet yours, or when a supersoft cat rubs up against your hand. A recent study found that men with AIDS were less likely to suffer from depression if they owned a pet.

Pets encourage you to get out and exercise.

Whether people walk their dogs because they need it or are more likely to enjoy a walk when they have companionship, dog owners do spend more time walking than non-pet owners, at least if they live in an urban setting. Because exercise is good for stress management and overall health, owning a dog can be credited with increasing these benefits.

Pets can help with social support.

When we're out walking, having a dog with us can make us more approachable and give people a reason to stop and talk, thereby increasing the number of people we meet. This gives us an opportunity to increase our network of friends and acquaintances, which also provides great stress-management benefits.

Pets control blood pressure better than drugs do.

While ACE-inhibitor drugs (angiotensin-converting-enzyme inhibitor) generally reduce blood pressure, they aren't as effective at controlling spikes in blood pressure due to stress and tension. However, in a study on pets and blood pressure, groups of hypertensive New York stockbrokers who adopted dogs or cats were found to have lower blood pressure and heart rates than those who didn't have pets. When the non-pet group heard about the results, most of them went out and got pets!

Pets can reduce stress more than people do.

While we all know the power of talking about your problems with a good friend who's also a good listener, spending time with a pet may be even better! One study showed that when people are conducting a task that's stressful, they experienced less stress when their pets were with them than when a supportive friend or even their spouse was present! (This may be partially due to the fact that pets don't judge us, they just love us unconditionally.)

Pets stave off loneliness and provide unconditional love.

Pets can be there for you in ways that people can't. They can offer love and companionship, enjoy comfortable silences, can keep secrets, and are excellent snugglers. They can be the best antidote to loneliness. In fact, one study found that nursing home residents reported less loneliness when visited by dogs alone than when they spent time with dogs and other people! All these benefits can reduce the amount of stress people experience in response to feelings of social isolation and lack of social support.

Of course, owning a pet isn't for everyone. They do come with additional work and responsibility, which can bring its own stress. However, for most people, the benefits of having a pet outweigh the drawbacks. Having a furry best friend can reduce stress in your life and bring you support when times get tough.

Meditation and Deep Breathing

One of the hardest things to do correctly is something we do every day (and often take for granted). Breathing is something all of us do all the time, yet most of us don't do it effectively. Stop and pay attention to your breathing right now. Do you see anything moving? If not, it is likely because you are taking shallow breaths. To really benefit your health, you should take long, deep breaths.

Deep breathing should be a part of our everyday lives. It not only can lengthen the time we get to live, but can also make us happier, more productive, and more energetic while living. Breathing deeply is a well-known stress reliever and offers a multitude of health benefits. In our high-stress, busy lives, we often breathe shallowly, but with a little effort, deep breathing can become an easy and unconscious part of our daily lives. By making a conscious decision to focus on our breath for a part of each day, we can breathe more deeply without having to think about it at all.

Spend some time each day consciously breathing slowly and rhythmically and bringing air down deeper into your lungs. It is a simple trick to automatically get you energized and focused. Picture your lungs expanding with air as you breathe in. That is exactly what happens. Shallow breathing only fills a small portion of your lungs, but it is so much healthier and more beneficial for all of your body's processes, systems and organs, to fill the lungs and bring air deep down into them. Doing this drives more oxygen into the body, which cleanses the blood and in turn cleanses and benefits everything else.

Breathe deeply into your abdomen, not just your chest. Proper breathing should be deep, slow, and rhythmic, and done through the nose, not the mouth. Each breath should ideally last three to four seconds breathing in, and three to four seconds breathing out. Deep, full breaths that fill your lungs use your diaphragm. When you breathe deeply, your diaphragm muscle pulls your lungs down, so they expand, and you can circulate oxygen down into the whole lung.

Breathe in slowly, and imagine your lungs filling up with air: your chest slightly widens, your diaphragm pulls your chest cavity down, and your belly button pulls away from your spine as you breathe in. When your lungs are full, exhale slowly and pull your belly button back in toward your spine to push out all the air.

Breathing deeply for just a few minutes every day will improve your mental outlook as well as your physical health. Breathing is something we all have to do anyway. Learn to do it well and make it a habit so you do it unconsciously, and you will be happier and healthier, and possibly even live longer.

Try this simple exercise: Breathe in and count to five while you draw the air in through your nose deep into your lungs. Hold for three seconds and release slowly through your mouth for five seconds. Visualize smelling flowers and blowing out candles.

11 Benefits of Deep Breathing

1. **Deep breathing relieves pain.** Studies have proven this, yet when you feel pain, your immediate unconscious reaction is to hold your breath. Remember that breathing deeply and breathing into pain will help you to release it. Deep breathing releases endorphins, which are the body's natural feel-good painkillers.

2. **Deep breathing makes you happier.** Breathing deeply increases neurochemical production in your brain and releases more of the chemicals that elevate moods and control pain.

3. **Deep breathing makes you calmer.** Breathing deeply and feeling calm is your natural state. Deep breathing naturally relaxes your mind and body. Breathing deeply is the fastest way to stimulate your parasympathetic nervous system, otherwise known as the relaxation response, which makes you feel relaxed. Stress is at the core of most diseases, and most of us live stressful, busy lives, which are commonly accompanied by shallow breathing. This means the body does not receive as much oxygen as it needs, and it makes your muscles constrict. You can almost feel this tightening when you are stressed or tense. When we feel stress or anxiety, the sympathetic nervous system is triggered and sends out spikes of cortisol and adrenaline. The parasympathetic nervous system counteracts this. Breathing is the fastest way for these two systems to communicate. With deeper breathing, you can turn the switch from high alarm to low in seconds. So, if you ever feel anxious, breathe deeply. Pay attention and you can feel the peace coming in and the tension being released as you simply (but deeply) breathe in and out.

4. **Deep breathing helps to detoxify your body.** Our bodies are designed to release 70% of their toxins through breathing. Carbon dioxide is a natural toxic waste that comes from the body's metabolic processes, and it needs to be expelled from the body regularly and consistently. It gets transferred from the blood to our

lungs, and we expel it with every breath. However, when our lungs are compromised by shallow breathing, the other detoxification systems in the body take over and have to work harder to expel this waste. This overload can make the body weaker and lead to illness.

5. **Deep breathing gives you energy.** Drawing air deeper down into the lungs greatly increases blood flow, as this is where the greatest amount of blood flow occurs, according to the American Medical Student Association. This increases energy and improves stamina. The higher oxygen content of the blood, which cleanses the body and all its cells of debris and toxins, along with better circulation, better sleep, stress reduction, your body working more efficiently, and all that goes along with these naturally gives you lots more energy.

6. **Deep breathing helps to improve your posture.** Bad posture is often directly linked to incorrect breathing. Try it yourself, and as you practice breathing deeply, watch how you naturally straighten up. Filling your lungs encourages you to straighten your spine and stand or sit taller.

7. **Deep breathing increases your cardiovascular capacity.** It can enhance the benefits you get from exercise. Aerobic exercise (cardio) uses fat as energy, while anaerobic exercise (strength training) uses glucose as energy. By expanding your cardiovascular capacity from deep breathing, you can do more cardio activities more easily, which also increases your cardiovascular capacity and burns more fat cells.

8. **Deep breathing stimulates the lymphatic system.** The lymphatic system is a crucial system in your body that most of us are unaware of. We have twice the amount of lymphatic fluid in our body as we do blood. Our circulatory system relies on our heart to pump it, while the lymphatic system relies on our breathing to get it moving. Blood pumps oxygen and nutrients to cells and, once they absorb what they need, they excrete their waste back out into the sea of lymphatic fluid that our cells constantly swim in. The lymphatic fluid is responsible for ridding the body of the debris the cells excrete, along with dead cells and other waste. Because our breathing is what moves the lymph, breathing shallowly can lead to a sluggish lymphatic system that does not detoxify properly. Deep breathing will help get that lymph flowing properly so your body can work more efficiently.

9. **Deep breathing helps to regulate weight.** If you are underweight, the extra oxygen will help to feed the cells and tissues. If you are overweight, it will assist with weight loss. The extra oxygen in the body will help to burn up excess fat more efficiently. When you are stressed, your body tends to burn glycogen instead of fat. Deep breathing triggers the relaxation response, which encourages the body to burn fat instead.

10. **Deep breathing improves your digestion.** More oxygen is supplied to the digestive organs, thereby helping them to work more efficiently. Deeper breathing also increases blood flow, which encourages intestinal action in the digestive tract and further improves your overall digestion. In addition, deeper

breathing results in a calmer nervous system, which in turn enhances optimal digestion.

11. **Deep breathing strengthens your major organs, such as lungs and heart.** Deep breathing expands the lungs and makes them work more efficiently. It also brings more oxygen to the blood, which gets sent to the heart so that the heart does not have to work so hard to deliver oxygen to tissues. Also, with the lungs working a little harder pushing oxygen out into the blood, it eases the pressure needed by the heart to pump it through the body. This improves your circulation and gives the heart a bit of a break.

Deep breathing improves overall health and lowers your chances of sickness or disease.

Deep breathing helps you sleep better.

Deep breathing lowers your blood pressure.

Deep breathing is one of the easiest ways to improve your health dramatically, and you can do it anywhere, at any time. It costs nothing and takes very little effort. Take a little time each day to practice breathing deeply, and your efforts will be rewarded.

As you can see, regular exercise and proper nutrition are not only good for the body, they are also the most effective ways to improve your mental health. While it's true that a solid exercise and nutrition regimen can improve your physical health, trim your waistline, and even add years to your life, that's not what motivates most people to stay active. People who exercise regularly tend to do so because it gives them an enormous sense of well-being. They feel more energetic throughout the day, sleep better at night, have sharper memories, and feel more relaxed and positive about themselves and their lives.

But just as important as all that new-found energy is getting proper rest and recovery. Let's address that in the next chapter.

CHAPTER 6

REST AND RECOVERY

The human body was not designed to sit—it was designed for movement. Although exercise is a major component of staying healthy, so too are rest and recovery. The most important aspect of rest is sleep. Adequate levels of sleep help to provide better mental health, hormonal balance, and muscular recovery. Also important is recovery, which refers to techniques and actions taken to maximize your body's repair. Critical actions here include hydration, good posture, stretching, and again, as a recurring theme, proper nutrition.

Recovery from Activity and Exercise

So, you started your New Year's resolutions, one of which no doubt was to get healthy and fit in the upcoming year! You spent time planning your workout, but did you stop and think about your recovery plan? Whether you're new to exercise or just changing up your routine, proper recovery after a workout is just as critical as the workout itself.

Is recovery really that important?

In a word, yes! When you exercise, you put your body through a controlled amount of stress and understand that stress is essential for your tissues to improve their function and for adequate performance. What actually happens is that you get microtears in your muscles from the imposed demand of your activity. So, recovery gives you a chance to build yourself back up, so you are stronger than before. It is, in essence, the link between your short-term (immediate) benefits and long-term (lasting) outcome.

Here are some strategies to help you gain maximum benefit from your workout while diminishing your risk of developing injuries.

Refueling (Nutrition and Hydration)

You may often take the initiative to make sure you properly nourish your body before exercising in order to optimize performance, but nutrition for recovery is often overlooked. When your tissues have been stressed during exercise, your body counts on a well-balanced variety of vitamins, minerals, and nutrients to assist in rebuilding and repairing those stressed areas. Including a healthy combination of proteins, carbs, and healthy fats will maximize the benefits of your efforts.

Don't forget about water! Proper hydration after exercise is extremely important for replacing the fluids you lost during your workout. Water is also crucial for maintaining healthy joints, regulating temperature, and eliminating wastes that build up in your system during exercise. It's always a good habit to keep a water bottle with you for easy, reliable access, whether it be in your gym bag, purse, car, or office.

Stretching

We know how important a role stretching plays in recovery, yet we rarely give it the time or attention it deserves. The reason you stretch is so you can maintain the flexibility of tissues that are stiff or tight from an activity or a prolonged position. It is important to distinguish between the two types of stretches we can perform—static and dynamic. Static stretching is when you hold a stretch for a prolonged period of time (such as a runner's stretch for your calf when you lean against a wall) and should be performed after exercising. Dynamic stretching is when you combine muscle groups by using movement (think hip circles, walking lunges, or butt kicks), and should be done prior to your workout.

For some individuals, stretching in addition to a workout is extravagant—a nice touch, but not really necessary. Or maybe you're the type of person who thinks that touching your toes for a few seconds after getting off the treadmill is plenty. But as it turns out, when and how you stretch your muscles can actually make or break your fitness goals.

Just Get Moving

Stretching before a workout is critical for preventing injury as well as improving performance. This is especially true if you exercise right after waking up or if you're fairly sedentary during the day, because your muscles will most likely be tight. Stretching for 15 minutes before a workout can help people avoid injury.

Exactly what type of stretching are we talking about here? We are talking about doing a dynamic warm-up before exercise. This is different from static stretches, which are typically held for 20–30 seconds in the same position (think hamstring stretches). A dynamic warm-up involves active movements that mimic your actual workout. If you've ever noticed runners getting ready for a race, they are most likely performing dynamic stretches such as hip circles, walking lunges, and butt kicks to activate the muscle groups used in running.

During dynamic stretching you are constantly moving, so it provides a cardio warm-up as well. Not only will you decrease your risk of injury, but dynamic stretching can help to improve athletic performance. It stands to reason that dynamic stretching enhances muscle performance and power output more than static stretching.

The Problem with Holding Tight

Because the thought of performing a mini-workout before your actual workout sounds exhausting, many of you instead resort to a few half-hearted toe touches after exercise. Static stretches, like these, focus more on relaxing muscles and promoting flexibility than dynamic stretching does, which is why static stretching is better to add to the end of your workout.

Recent research questioned the benefits of static stretching before a workout, suggesting it may lead to decreased athletic performance. One study found that performing static stretches before doing a barbell squat caused individuals to feel off-balance and lift less weight. Another study showed that soccer players who performed static stretches before a 30-meter sprint had slower times than players who did not stretch beforehand.

Here's another bummer: Some research suggests that stretching won't do much to eliminate muscle soreness. In a review of 12 studies, researchers found that pre- or post-exercise stretching did not stop troublesome aches and pains. The likely reason? Microtears in the muscle and surrounding connective tissue, which stretching won't repair, are to blame for soreness.

The Bottom Line

So, what's the conclusion? Perform dynamic stretches before a workout, which can prepare your muscles and even improve athletic performance. With all the evidence against it, it's probably wise to avoid static stretches before a workout. But static stretches can certainly be helpful if you spend a lot of time sitting at a desk. Loosen up shoulders, back muscles, hip flexors, and hamstrings with static stretches (post-workout) a few times a week. But your BEST bet is to have a physical therapist design a program tailored to your individual goals and abilities. You will thank them when you are injury-free for years to come!

Cross-Training

Cross-training allows you to challenge your body with different tasks to make sure that certain tissues do not get overstressed (which can lead to injuries). Try a variety of different exercises, which could include running, walking, cycling, swimming, weightlifting, yoga, or Pilates. And don't simply do exercises that you like to do (although this is important for motivation and sticking with your program)—do exercises that your body needs. This is where a physical therapist can help you discover whether you are prone to overuse injuries by determining any deficiencies in your workout regimen.

Workout injuries can often be attributed to excessive repetition of the same activity. The body tends to wear down when subjected to the same motions over and over again, placing an incredible amount of stress on ligaments, joints, tendons, and muscles. Cross-training allows the overused portions of your body to rest. As for recovery, cross-training improves conditioning, reduces the odds of injury, and even hastens the recovery period by boosting blood flow. Improved blood flow transmits nutrients to damaged muscle tissues, allowing for faster recovery.

Listen to Your Body

Nobody knows how your body feels after a workout better than you do. But you must recognize the signs of fatigue, pain, or discomfort so you can adjust recovery time between workouts. This could also include pushing yourself to work harder when you are feeling well.

And for heaven's sake, don't worry about what others are doing at the gym! Trust in yourself and the signs your body is giving you. Don't ever be reluctant to ask your physical therapist for some tips on how your body may give you feedback after exercise, as well as the best ways to respond.

Get Enough Sleep

I'm sure many of you have heard a colleague or coworker say, "Sleep is overrated!" Sleep is your body's premier opportunity to repair and recover, yet it is often taken for granted. According to the Centers for Disease Control and Prevention (CDC), adults should get 7 to 8 hours of sleep each night, while teens should get 9 to 10 hours.

These guidelines take on greater significance when you are exercising and demanding more of your body (or perform stressful daily activities). When you sleep, your cardiovascular, muscular, skeletal, and immune systems can begin their repair processes. To get the most benefits from a restful sleep, avoid stimulating activities while in bed (such as watching TV or using your smartphone) and strive for consistent bedtimes.

Plan Ahead

Yes, life gets hectic! It's very easy to get caught up in the hustle and bustle of daily life and neglect your needs in the process. Don't let your health suffer when the unexpected comes up. Plan your day (or week) so you have ample time to work out, and to follow and implement the strategies listed throughout this book. This way, you won't feel as rushed and possibly miss out on important recovery activities.

Good Sleep Habits

We spend almost 1/3 of our lives sleeping, yet we still struggle to make sleep a priority—it really makes no sense. You'll find quality healthcare tips for keeping you healthy and mobile, understanding why it's important to take care of your body, and knowing when and how to deal with discomfort to your neck, back, shoulder, knee, wrist, ankle, so you can continue to enjoy the activities you love.

But the one thing that is simple and free and can pay immediate dividends to your overall health is to get quality sleep! Quality sleep just might be the most important thing you do each day.

If you search for information regarding sleep in newspaper or magazine articles or browse the internet, you'll see that sleep is one of the things all healthcare professionals agree on. They might disagree about things like what should go on your plate for an ideal diet, or the best workout routine to burn calories, but if there's one topic they can all agree on it is sleep, and with very good reason.

I have yet to confer with a nutritionist, dietician, or other healthcare expert who suggests that the best way to achieve optimum health is by sleeping less or not getting quality sleep! But guess what? That's exactly what many of you do too often! So, what happens when you don't get enough sleep? You gain weight, your stress level increases, your potential for injury increases—and those are just for starters. Does this sound like the outcome you are actively seeking? I think not!

Let's look at some things that happen when you don't get enough sleep. First, as I briefly touched on above, lack of quality sleep is strongly linked to weight gain. As you sleep your body is repaired, and hormone levels are rebalanced. By not getting enough sleep, your body is put under stress, which prompts the "fight or flight" response. This tends to cause a hormonal imbalance, which in turn often leads to weight gain, since your body is "out of whack." Hormonal imbalances can also disrupt the feelings that you are either hungry or full. By not getting enough sleep, hunger levels go up—and the feeling you get when you are full will be lessened. This tends to make you feel hungrier than if you were well rested. So, if you're always feeling hungry and never seem to be satisfied, ask yourself whether you're getting enough sleep!

Quality sleep also plays a large role in your physical health, as it is involved in healing and repairing your blood vessels and your heart. Ongoing sleep deficiency is linked to an increased risk of heart disease, kidney disease, high blood pressure, diabetes, and even stroke.

Ever get mood swings? Lack of sleep could be the culprit! Feelings of irritability, impatience, and inability to concentrate may be traced back to a lack of sleep. This is certainly not someone I would choose to be around!

I started off this section by stating that we spend almost 1/3 of our lives sleeping. So why do we have such difficulty making sleep a priority? Because if something is not a priority, it becomes awfully difficult to fix if we have no clue where to begin!

I'm sure many of you reading this are under the assumption that going to bed early is a good thing. After all, didn't Ben Franklin say, "Early to bed and early to rise makes a man healthy, wealthy, and wise"? Only thing is, I'm fairly sure Ben didn't consider TV in his wisdom! Getting into bed and turning on the TV is not the way to get quality sleep (despite thinking that you are just "winding down").

What is Quality Sleep?

There are four key determinants of quality sleep, as published in a report by Sleep Health.

- Sleeping more time while in bed (at least 85% of the total time)
- Falling asleep within 30 minutes or less
- Waking up no more than once per night
- Being awake for 20 minutes or less after initially falling asleep

Here are some things that will help you get quality sleep.

Sleep on a good-quality mattress. Make sure your mattress is comfortable and supportive. The one you have been using for years may have exceeded its life expectancy, which is generally eight years for most good-quality mattresses.

Evaluate your room. Your bedroom should be cool (between 60 and 67 degrees), as well as free from any noise or light that could disturb your sleep. Consider using blackout curtains, an eye mask, ear plugs, a white noise machine, humidifier, fan, or other devices.

Stick to a sleep schedule. This means going to bed and waking up at the same time every day, including weekends. This helps to regulate your body's clock and could help you fall asleep and stay asleep.

Practice a relaxing bedtime ritual. A relaxing, routine activity right before bedtime and away from bright lights helps to separate your sleep time from activities that can cause stress, anxiety, or excitement, which make it more difficult to fall asleep, get sound and deep sleep, and remain asleep.

Exercise daily. Vigorous exercise is best, but any activity is better than no activity. Exercise at any time of day, but not at the expense of your sleep.

Avoid alcohol, cigarettes, and heavy meals in the evening. These can all disrupt sleep. Eating large or spicy meals can cause discomfort from indigestion. If possible, avoid eating big meals for two to three hours before bedtime. If you're still hungry, eat a light snack 45 minutes before bedtime.

Wind down. Your body needs time to shift into sleep mode, so try and spend the last hour before bedtime doing a calming activity such as reading. For some individuals, using an electronic device such as an iPad or phone can make it hard to fall asleep, because the blue light emanating from the screens activates the brain.

If you can't fall asleep, go into another room and do something relaxing until you feel tired. It's a good idea to remove work materials, TVs, and computers from the sleeping environment. Your bed should only be used for two things—sleep and sex. This will help strengthen the association between bed and sleep. If you associate a particular activity or item with anxiety about sleeping, remove it from your bedtime routine.

If you're still having difficulty sleeping, consider a consult with a sleep professional. You may also benefit from keeping a sleep journal (or diary) to help you better evaluate common issues or patterns with your sleeping habits.

So, make quality sleep a priority! It is extremely important for your health, and best of all, it's absolutely free! I understand that quite often life gets in the way. You spend time with your children or grandchildren during the day, leaving the evening as your only "me" time. In the long run, the extra hours of sleep will reward you as you'll be happier, more patient, and more alert during the day, leaving you with tons more energy to do the things you love and enjoy.

Best and Worst Sleeping Positions

If you've ever heard someone say, "sleep is overrated," think again! For something we spend up to 1/3 of our lives doing, it's not such a simple thing. Both sleeping too much and sleeping too little have been linked to a number of health problems, from obesity and heart disease to dementia and diabetes. Furthermore, sleep can play a role in snoring, heartburn, and even wrinkles!

Here are your choices of sleep positions from best to worst, complete with pros and cons. I'll leave it up to you to decide which is best for you.

Sleeping on Your Back

Pros: The majority of doctors agree this is the best sleeping position, especially for neck and spine health, because the back is straight and not forced into any contortions. This position also helps the mattress do its intended job of supporting the spine. In a perfect (and most likely uncomfortable) world, you would sleep on your back without a pillow, since this position leaves the neck in a neutral alignment. Using too many pillows, however, may make breathing more difficult. Back sleepers don't have their faces smooshed up against pillows, so this may actually lead to fewer facial wrinkles. And for anyone suffering from neck pain, simply rolling up a towel and inserting it into your pillowcase can provide much needed support. Similarly, for those of you with lower back pain, rolling up a blanket and placing it under your knees can help you get the restful sleep you may be lacking.

Cons: Snoring and episodes of sleep apnea are much more common when you sleep on your back. In fact, if you have been diagnosed with sleep apnea, then sleeping on your side is the preferred sleep position. When you sleep on your back, gravity forces the base of the tongue to collapse into the airway, leading to obstructed breathing and snoring.

Sleeping on Your Side

Pros: Whether curled up in a fetal position or lying straight on one side, this position seems to be the most popular! Doctors encourage expectant mothers to sleep on their left sides during pregnancy since it improves circulation to the heart. Side sleeping is also encouraged during pregnancy, since sleeping on your back can increase pressure on your lower back due to the added weight, and sleeping on your stomach is, well, impractical for obvious reasons.

For men and those of you not expecting, sleeping on the left side can also help to ease acid reflux and heartburn, making it easier for them to doze off.

Cons: Sleeping on the left side can increase pressure on the stomach and lungs, so alternate sides to prevent organ strain. Also, side sleepers often awaken with pins and needles in the arms they've been lying on, since resting the head (or the whole body) on a single arm can restrict blood flow and compress nerves. In this position, a lot of stress is placed on the shoulders, leading to possible tightening and constriction of the neck and shoulder muscles.

Sleeping on Your Stomach

Pros: Sleeping on your stomach limits your chances of snoring and, in some cases, can ease sleep apnea. However, that's pretty much it for the benefits!

Cons: Sleeping on your stomach is generally regarded as the worst sleeping position. It reduces and flattens the natural curve of your spine, potentially leading to increased back pain. Sleeping all night with your head turned to one side is not good for your neck either.

However, if this happens to be your preferred sleeping position, try using pillows to gradually train your body to sleep on one side. If you start to experience lower back discomfort, try putting a pillow under your hips and lower abdomen to help support the base of your spine and keep the natural curve in your lower back from flattening out.

So, what's the verdict?

Individuals tend to sleep in the positions they find most comfortable, regardless of health benefits. There's no harm in experimenting with different sleeping positions, so feel free to try each position for a couple of nights to see which is the best fit for you. Whether it's back, side, or stomach, people tend to awaken in the position that their bodies naturally snooze in. Unless a doctor or physical therapist specifically recommends switching, it's probably best to keep doing what feels right for you.

Insomnia

If you have difficulty sleeping, you may be wondering whether you have insomnia, which is the most common sleep disorder in the United States. The National Institutes of Health estimates that approximately 30% of the general population suffers from sleep disruption, and around 10% has associated symptoms of daytime functional impairment. This is generally described as difficulty falling asleep or staying asleep, even when an individual has the chance to do so. People with insomnia often feel dissatisfied with their sleep, and often experience one or more of the following symptoms:

- Difficulty falling asleep
- Difficulty staying asleep (waking up during the night and not being able to get back to sleep)
- Waking up too early in the morning
- Not feeling refreshed upon awaking (known as nonrestorative sleep)
- Experiencing low energy or fatigue during the day
- Mood swings, which can lead to irritability
- Cognitive impairment, such as difficulty concentrating
- Behavior problems, such as feeling aggressive or impulsive
- Difficulty at school or work
- Difficulty with personal relationships, including family, friends, and caregivers

How long does insomnia last?

Insomnia is characterized based on duration—acute or chronic. Acute insomnia tends to be short-lasting and is often associated with life circumstances. Have you ever lied awake at night, staring at the ceiling and wishing you could fall asleep? This can be due to receiving stressful news, starting a new job, experiencing jet lag, or the night before an exam, for instance. Acute insomnia tends to be fairly common and often resolves itself without treatment.

Chronic insomnia is sleep disruption that occurs at least three nights per week and lasts at least three months. There may be numerous causes at work here, including unhealthy sleep habits, changes in the environment, shift work, and certain medications. Chronic insomnia tends to be associated with comorbidity, meaning it is linked to another medical or psychiatric issue.

The question becomes: How do you distinguish a normal, passing sleep problem from a more serious form of insomnia that requires treatment?

Let's take a closer look at some factors that can cause chronic insomnia. One such factor involves medical causes. There can be a direct cause (the medical condition itself causes insomnia) or an indirect cause (the medical condition causes discomfort, which makes falling asleep difficult). Some examples of medical conditions that can cause insomnia are…

- Arthritis
- Asthma
- Chronic pain
- Endocrine problems (such as hypo/hyperthyroidism)
- Gastrointestinal problems (such as acid reflux)
- Low-back pain
- Nasal or sinus allergies
- Neurological conditions (such as Parkinson's disease)

Medications taken for asthma, birth control, depression, heart disease, high blood pressure, nasal allergies and the common cold, and thyroid disease can also cause insomnia.

Insomnia may also be a symptom of underlying sleep disorders, such as sleep apnea or restless legs syndrome. It can also be caused by psychiatric conditions such as depression. Psychological struggles can make sleeping difficult, and insomnia itself can bring on mood changes and hormonal shifts. It is important to understand that symptoms of depression, such as loss of interest or motivation, low energy, and feelings of sadness or hopelessness, can be linked with insomnia, and one can make the other worse. There is good news, however—both are treatable, regardless of which came first.

Most individuals have experienced difficulty sleeping at some point due to anxiety—feeling worried or nervous. Some symptoms of anxiety that can lead to insomnia include…

- Feeling of tension
- Being revved up or overstimulated
- Excessive worrying about future events
- Feeling overwhelmed by responsibilities
- Getting caught up in thoughts about past events

In addition, anxiety can be associated with onset insomnia (difficulty falling asleep) or maintenance insomnia (waking during the night and not being able to get back to sleep). In either instance, the quiet and inactivity of night often causes stressful thoughts or fears, which keep the person awake.

Insomnia can also be caused by unhealthy lifestyles and sleep patterns.

- You may sleep in late some days to make up for lost sleep. But this can confuse your body's clock and make falling asleep at night more difficult.
- You take naps during the day (even if they're short ones). While short naps may be beneficial to some, they may make it more difficult to fall asleep at night for others.
- You bring work home with you and do it in the evening. This can certainly make it difficult to unwind and may cause you to feel preoccupied when it comes time to go to sleep. The blue light emitted from your computer may also make your brain more alert.

- You are working different shifts. Nontraditional hours can confuse your body's clock, especially if you are attempting to sleep during the day, or if your schedule changes from time to time.

Certain substances and activities, including eating patterns, may contribute to insomnia.

- **Caffeine** is a stimulant. In moderation, it can be fine for many people. But it can stay in your system for as long as eight hours, so the effects can be long-lasting. If you have difficulty sleeping, do not consume food, or drinks with caffeine, too close to bedtime.
- **Nicotine** is also a stimulant. As with caffeine, smoking tobacco products close to bedtime can make it hard to fall asleep and to get restful sleep. I don't need to warn anyone of the dangers of smoking!
- **Alcohol** is a sedative. It can make you fall asleep initially but may disrupt your sleep later in the night.
- **Heavy meals:** The best practice is to eat lightly before going to bed. Eating too much in the evening may cause discomfort and make it difficult for you to settle down and relax. In addition, eating spicy foods before going to sleep may lead to heartburn and indigestion, which can interfere with your sleep.

Diagnosing insomnia

To date, there is no definitive test for insomnia. Doctors use many different tools to diagnose and measure insomnia symptoms. Some of the more common ones are as follows:

Sleep log: This is simply a diary in which you keep track of details about your sleep. Here you will write down things such as the time you go to bed and wake up, and how sleepy you feel at certain times of the day.

Sleep inventory: This is an extensive questionnaire about your medical history, personal health, and sleep patterns.

Blood tests: These are often performed to rule out or confirm other underlying medical conditions such as thyroid problems, which can interrupt sleep in some individuals.

Sleep study: Medically known as a polysomnography, this is an overnight study to gather information about your nighttime sleep. You will be hooked up to an EEG (electroencephalography), which measures brain waves associated with the different stages of sleep. You will also be monitored for oxygen levels, body movements, and heart and breathing patterns. This is considered a noninvasive test and actually does have you sleep in a bed.

Am I likely to be diagnosed with insomnia?

Consider answering the following questions before you speak with a medical professional.

- Exactly what type of sleeping troubles am I experiencing? Am I having difficulty falling asleep, staying asleep, or waking up too early? How often is this occurring (how many nights per week)?
- Write down your sleep schedule. What time do you go to bed? What time do you wake up? Do you nap during the day?
- Do you have different bedtimes and wake-up times on the weekend? Does your work schedule require you to adjust your sleeping habits at all?
- Do you lie awake worrying or feeling anxious about tasks and responsibilities?

- What do you do when you can't get to sleep? (For example, do you get out of bed, watch TV, read, or work on your computer?) Has anything worked in the past to help you sleep?
- How long have you experienced difficulty sleeping? Is this something new, or have you had trouble sleeping for as long as you can remember?
- Do you have any medical conditions?
- Have you recently experienced any major changes to your life or any stressful events such as a new job, a move, a breakup, or financial troubles?
- What is your sleep environment like? Do you sleep alone or with a partner? Is your room quiet and dark? Is your bed comfortable? Do you have any disturbances during the night, such as young children or pets?

What are some treatment considerations for insomnia?

It is very important to seek help if your insomnia has become a pattern, or if you often feel tired or unrefreshed during the day and this interferes with your everyday life. (This is mainly in regard to chronic insomnia.) Start by addressing the issue with your doctor or physical therapist. They will guide you through the next steps, which may involve an assessment and further testing, or a referral to a sleep specialist. Your doctor or physical therapist will provide you with some basic information and resources about healthy sleep habits or discuss possible medical treatment options. Some of these suggestions may include the following:

Nonmedical treatments for insomnia (behavioral and cognitive)

Some behavioral and psychological techniques can be extremely helpful for treating insomnia. These include relaxation training, sleep restriction, stimulus control, and cognitive behavioral therapy.

Relaxation training (also known as progressive muscle relaxation) instructs you to systematically tighten and relax muscles in different areas of your body. This helps with overall calming, which can help to induce sleep. Some other forms of relaxation techniques include breathing exercises, mindfulness, meditation, and guided imagery (listening to audio recordings to help you fall asleep or to return to sleep).

Stimulus control helps you build an association between sleep and the bedroom by limiting the type of activities allowed in the bedroom. Going to bed only when you are sleepy and getting out of bed if you've been awake for 20 minutes or more would be examples of stimulus control. This assists in breaking an unhealthy association between the bedroom and wakefulness.

Sleep restriction involves a strict schedule of bedtimes and wake times, and limits time in bed to only when you are sleeping.

Cognitive behavioral therapy (CBT) includes behavioral changes such as keeping a set bedtime and wake-up time, getting out of bed if you have been awake for 20 minutes or more, and eliminating afternoon naps. But it also adds a cognitive (thinking) component by challenging unhealthy fears and beliefs around sleep by teaching rational positive thinking.

Medical treatments for insomnia

There are numerous types of sleep aids for insomnia, including over-the-counter (nonprescription) and prescription medications. Always consult with a medical professional before taking any type of sleep aid.

Major classes of prescription insomnia medications include benzodiazepine hypnotics (for example, Diazepam, Klonopin, Tranxene, Xanax, or Valium), non-benzodiazepine hypnotics (for example, Celexa, Cymbalta, Paxil, Prozac, or Zoloft), and melatonin receptor agonists (Hetlioz, Melitor, Rozerem, Thymanax, or Valdoxan).

What to do when you can't sleep

If you have difficulty falling asleep, staying asleep, or waking up too early, there are some ways to help with each of these patterns.

Tips for falling asleep

- Allow at least 30 minutes to wind down before getting into bed, where you do something relaxing like reading. You can also try dimming the lights for an hour or so before bedtime.
- Stop using electronic devices like phones, tablets, and laptops for at least 30 minutes before climbing into bed, as the blue light emitted from their screens can alert the brain, making it more difficult to fall asleep.
- Perform deep-breathing or relaxation exercises to calm your mind and body.
- If you're lying in bed and can't fall asleep within 20 minutes, get up and go to another part of the house to do a relaxing activity such as reading or listening to music. You want your bed to only conjure sleepy thoughts and feelings, so by lying in bed awake, you are creating an unhealthy link between your sleeping environment and wakefulness.
- Wake up at the same time each day (including weekends), even if you had a hard time falling asleep the night before and feel tired in the morning. This can

help adjust your body's clock and make it easier to fall asleep at night.

Tips for staying asleep throughout the night

- Practice deep-breathing exercises.
- Refrain from caffeine in the afternoon and evening and avoid alcohol close to bedtime. These can promote wake-ups during the night.
- Ensure that your sleeping environment is dark and quiet throughout the night. Use blackout shades to block streetlights, neighbors' outdoor lights, and early-morning daylight. A fan or a noise machine can help to block sounds.
- If you're lying in bed and can't fall back asleep within 20 minutes, do not stay in bed worrying about not sleeping. Get up and go to another part of the house to do a relaxing activity, like reading, with dim light.

Tips for avoiding waking up too early

- Practice deep-breathing exercises.
- Make sure your sleeping environment is dark and quiet throughout the night. Use blackout shades to block outdoor lights from houses or from the street, as well as early-morning light. Use earplugs, a fan, or a noise machine to block sounds.

Special considerations for women

Women are more likely than men to experience insomnia. In a recent National Sleep Foundation survey, 57% of women (vs 51% of men) said they experienced insomnia at least a few nights each week. Yet only 7% of the women reported receiving treatment for insomnia. Certain phases of the menstrual cycle, pregnancy, and menopause can contribute to women's sleep difficulties. While these biological changes sometimes disrupt sleep, unhealthy sleep habits can maintain the pattern. This is why keeping good sleep practices is extremely important for women.

In addition to general healthy sleep recommendations, here are some tips to help women improve their sleep:

- If you're going through menopause, and your insomnia is caused by hormonal fluctuations and hot flashes, keep your room temperature cool and comfortable (between 60 and 67 degrees). If you sweat during the night, have a change of pajamas, extra pillowcase, and glass of water by your bed.
- If you're pregnant and have difficulty sleeping, keep multiple pillows on hand during the night. Try sleeping on your side with one pillow at your back, another between your knees, and a third one in front of you to rest your arm on. Also make sure to restrict fluid intake during the evening.
- For many women, insomnia is linked to depression. While deep-breathing and relaxation exercises can be helpful, it is important to discuss your symptoms with your doctor.

Insomnia and older adults

True or false: As we get older, our sleep needs decline. If you answered true, you are caught up in the misconception that we don't need as much sleep as we age. Older adults need between seven and nine hours of sleep per night. However, it can be a challenge for adults 65 or older to stay asleep throughout the night. According to another National Sleep Foundation survey, 39% of older Americans (aged 65+) were more likely to say they wake up a lot during the night, compared to 33% of those between ages 50 and 54, 31% of those between 30 and 49, and 24% of those between 18 and 29.

Now contrast those results with those individuals who stated they got a good night's sleep. In this case, 60% of those 65 and older reported getting a good night's sleep every night or almost every night, as compared to 52% of those between 50 and 54, 44% of those between 30 and 49, and only 38% of those between 18 and 29. So, even though aging seems to make certain aspects of sleep more difficult, many older adults claim they still feel good during the day.

Certain biological changes make sleep more difficult as you get older. One example is the shift in circadian rhythm that older adults can experience, which causes them to become sleepy in the early evening and wake up too early in the morning. Is it any wonder that this survey by the National Sleep Foundation found that 64% of the adults in the 65+ age group considered themselves to be "morning" people?

As mentioned earlier, I pointed out medical conditions and other sleep disorders that could cause insomnia. Again, examples might be health issues such as gastrointestinal and respiratory problems that can disrupt sleep. Also noted here would be sleep apnea, in which an individual briefly (but repeatedly) stops breathing during sleep.

Again, do not take symptoms of insomnia lightly. If you regularly have trouble sleeping or feel fatigued or unrefreshed during the day, talk to your doctor, physical therapist, or other medical professional. Small changes in sleep habits like skipping naps (or changing the time of your naps), or simply cutting back on caffeine can help. If your insomnia is related to a medical or psychiatric condition, entrust your medical team to put an appropriate treatment plan in place.

I hope you now have a better appreciation of why rest and recovery are every bit as important as exercise and proper nutrition. Your growth-hormone levels, which assist in muscle recovery, are at their highest when you sleep. If you take nothing away from this chapter other than the importance of getting quality sleep, then you've significantly improved your health. Of course, increasing your ability to memorize information, concentrate more easily, regulate your appetite, and maintain healthier body functions are all pluses.

Even when you do everything "right," you can still benefit from the care and advice of a healthcare professional. Who do you turn to? In the next chapter, we'll discuss your options.

CHAPTER 7

YOUR ALL-STAR HEALTHCARE TEAM

I've spent a good portion of this book educating you about preventative strategies you can use to take control of your health. I've discussed exercise, nutrition, stress reduction, mental well-being, and rest and recovery. But you shouldn't have to do it alone. Hopefully, you have a strong support system of family and friends. Now add a professional healthcare team, and you've really got your bases covered!

In this chapter, I'll lay out my best advice for assembling a team of top-notch healthcare professionals, so you'll never have to make another uninformed decision about your health again!

Who Should You Have on Your All-Star Healthcare Team?

I'm sure you know the saying "Look out for number one!" But in today's healthcare world, it could not be more confusing. Every day, you are faced with decision after decision for a multitude of daily activities: what to wear, what to eat, when to exercise, how to prioritize work tasks…and the list goes on. Is it any wonder that you often forego making the important decisions, such as the ones involving your health?

More than likely, you have done this at some point—neglecting your health, thinking "It's not too bad…yet." Or "I'll give it another week" (after 6 months have passed already). Or "I don't have time to deal with it now." Have you ever considered enlisting a team of knowledgeable medical professionals who you could contact at any time with any issue, and who could help you make the best possible healthcare decisions while eliminating guesswork?

Consider for a second how vital a team is. After all, you never see a boxing match that didn't have a "corner," or a NASCAR driver who didn't have a pit crew. These teams are specifically trained to assess problems early or to fix them when they arise. Why should this level of proactive care happen only at these elite levels? You are entitled to be treated in this manner. Who would you want on your All-Star Healthcare Team?

When selecting members for your All-Star Team, a good question to ask a potential provider is "How much time will I actually be spending with you each visit?" Another question to ask is "Should a problem arise that needs immediate attention, what's the best way to contact you?" After all, your team should be accessible!   What's the point of having a team if you have to wait three or four weeks to see them?

Here are my recommendations for who you should have on your All-Star Healthcare Team.

Family Physician

A family doctor is one of your most vital team members. This person should be someone you trust immensely, as they are the gatekeepers for all your healthcare needs. This individual should be extremely knowledgeable and patient, and love to educate. This is your go-to person for all things related to medical illness who will keep your vital information handy, so any issues can be detected early.

Physicians are responsible for promoting, restoring, or maintaining health—very important! You will likely see your family doctor once or twice a year (if not more often). Sore throat? Stomach bug? Fever? Rapid and unexpected weight loss? Dip in energy level? Unresolved pain issue? These are just a few of the reasons a family physician should be a top person on your team!

Physical Therapist

Your physical therapist is a musculoskeletal and movement expert (think muscles, joints, bones, and nerves). In a nutshell, if it hurts when you move, then your physical therapist is the person to see. The added bonus of having a physical therapist on your All-Star Team is that in most states, anyone can see a physical therapist right away without having to get a referral from a physician, physician's assistant, nurse practitioner, or dentist—which is known as direct access.

Wilderman Physical Therapy is a direct access clinic. This is to our clients' advantage, as the majority of injuries are treated most effectively when we can see individuals immediately following the incidents.

Another significant bonus to having a go-to physical therapist on your team is the fact that a physical therapist's training spans a multitude of orthopaedic body systems.

Oftentimes, when we see a client for an initial assessment, they have already done quite a bit of research on their own or have consulted their family physician.

While a diagnosis from a family physician may be close, often the true mechanical issue requires more thorough examination. Sometimes a problem that appears to be a herniated disc, for example, may actually just be an issue of muscular-tissue or nerve-tissue tension. This is truly where the physical therapist's expertise is most valuable.

We are able to look at the entire movement picture and determine the true underlying cause of the problem rather than basing our findings on the symptoms alone. This gives our clients long-lasting relief and the best chances at recovery, so their issues do not reoccur.

Do you go to your family physician for an annual physical regardless of whether you have any medical issues? Do you see your dentist twice a year for a cleaning and checkup, even if you have no issues with your teeth? Do you see your auto mechanic every 3,000 to 5,000 miles for an oil change, even if your car is running smoothly?

But how many of you see a physical therapist on a yearly basis for a "full body tune-up?" Very few, I'm guessing, if any! Wouldn't it make sense for you to get screened by a musculoskeletal expert to make sure you remain pain-free? This way, we could address any possible areas of breakdown and resolve any potential issues that may escalate to more serious problems down the road.

Clients nowadays are becoming much savvier regarding their healthcare. Most of my clients ask tremendously insightful questions about the particular issues they are dealing with. Never hesitate to ask questions of your physical therapist or family physician. Those of us who truly value the client education experience enjoy explaining our methods to people who express an interest. And anytime either your physical therapist or family physician does not have adequate time to educate you about your healthcare, it may be time to find a new one!

Another factor that sets All-Star physical therapists and family physicians apart is that we stay in close contact with our clients. That way, if any future questions arise, you can easily reach us by phone, text, or email and will receive a quick and timely response. How many of you have that relationship with your physical therapist or family physician?

The key to be a great advocate for yourself is to do the research—that is, find out what makes the physical therapist you are going to see exceptional! It's no different than when you're looking for a family physician, dentist, auto mechanic, or surgeon. Do you truly want the best, or will you settle for "good enough"?

And once you've found your All-Star physical therapist, make sure your family physician and other medical professionals on your team know who they should be partnering with to ensure you are treated in the best possible way. At Wilderman Physical Therapy, our clients become better advocates for themselves because they are armed with the knowledge to treat themselves or to consult with a member of their team.

Specialist Physician

You may encounter a medical issue that needs more detailed attention or a deeper knowledge of a particular body system (such as heart, lungs, kidneys, joints, or nerves). These specialists exist due to their superior level of knowledge in their particular area. This makes them better qualified to assess and treat medical issues.

In addition, many of these specialists are also surgeons, should the need for surgery arise. A great orthopaedic surgeon, for example, will not tell you that you need surgery initially. If an orthopaedic condition can be treated conservatively (thus avoiding surgery), then this is the route they will recommend. This is how physical therapists and surgeons have developed such amazing relationships with their clients over history.

Unfortunately, there are still way too many physicians out there who don't understand the difference between physical therapy clinics and physical therapists. Their understanding is very similar to what the general public thinks: that all physical therapy is the same, regardless of whether you go to Wilderman Physical Therapy or to a large "mill-like" physical therapy clinic where they treat four to five clients at the same time. Nothing could be further from the truth!

Dentist

All right—this one is a gimme! There is simply no other medical profession that can take care of your teeth like they do. Got tooth pain? Want to keep your teeth pearly white? Make sure you have a great dentist on your All-Star Team!

There is, however, some overlap between the dental and physical therapy professions, especially when it comes to jaw pain and potential headaches related to TMJ (temporomandibular joint) issues. Beware the dentist who tells you that you simply need to wear a night guard or bite plate while you sleep to avoid grinding your teeth at night. While this may be beneficial, it's only part of the solution.

Since TMJ issues involve the jaw and not the teeth, many TMJ sufferers benefit tremendously from seeing a skilled physical therapist who is trained in manual therapy for soft tissue (muscles, tendons, ligaments) and joints associated with the face, jaw, and neck, which are the culprits in referring pain to the jaw and teeth.

Alternative/Complimentary Disciplines

Many professionals, including chiropractors, acupuncturists, massage therapists, personal trainers, dietitians, and nutritionists, fit into this category. Having one or more of these professionals on your All-Star Team would certainly bolster it. I have developed relationships with a number of individuals in this category who I can consult with to co-treat patients for the best possible outcomes.

Another reason you want the best physical therapist to oversee your healthcare needs

Many individuals nowadays use personal trainers or strength coaches to help them excel at sports and other activities. What great members to have on your team! But be very careful that your skills expert is aware of any movement or functional issues that may be preventing you from performing a particular drill or exercise with correct technique.

Think of those people who are specifically training in rotary sports—baseball players, softball players, golfers, and those who play any sport involving throwing. Oftentimes, I will hear "My coach wants me to be able to do this drill, but no matter how many times we work on it, I just can't seem to improve." This is a huge red flag, a dead giveaway that this person's body is simply not allowing them to perform the task. It has nothing to do with their motivation to do it correctly. They obviously have a compensation movement pattern that, if left unaddressed, will most likely lead to injury.

There you have it. You now have my recommendations for assembling your All-Star Healthcare Team. Keep in mind that you may never have to use some of these professionals, most notably in the specialist physician and alternative or complimentary disciplines. But it is certainly worth identifying these individuals in case a need should arise. That way you are being proactive with your healthcare instead of waiting until you need one of these individuals immediately!

Now that you've identified the valuable members to include on your All-Star Team, you must know who you do **not** want making healthcare decisions on your behalf: your insurance company! Most individuals I know talk about their health insurance the same way they talk about a friend who nobody likes. And believe me—you really don't see what's going on behind the scenes. If your health insurance was so great, you would have an accessible doctor who didn't make you wait and had plenty of time to spend with you.

Please realize this important point—no matter how much you pay for health insurance premiums, the medical professionals delivering your services are still restricted in the amount of time and scope of service they can offer you, because the insurance company will ultimately decide what will be covered. This can be frustrating for the professional who simply wants to help you!

Another thing I hear from clients is "I think my insurance is pretty good." Well, if their insurance was so good, why are their doctor visits getting shorter and shorter? Here's my answer: Your well-intentioned physician reports to your insurance that they saw you on a given day and notes the reason for the visit. Then your insurance company almost always counters with a denial! This is their first line of defense for not having to pay out.

Sadly, this one tactic is enough to dissuade some medical professionals from seeking reimbursement for that particular service. The problem is that after enough denials, some professionals will simply stop offering that service for fear of the long and tedious process required to recover their due reimbursement, regardless of how effective or important that service is for your care.

This happens every day in large "mill-like" physical therapy clinics that work in sheer volume. Their treatments may no longer be dictated by what you need or what's in your best interest for recovery, but sadly by which procedures your insurance company will reimburse them for. And it will only continue to get worse, as every day, third-party reimbursement continues to decrease while insurance premiums continue to increase.

The point I'm trying to make here is simple—insurance companies are looking out for profits, not for your well-being! As long as this continues, you are going to see lower quality care and higher volumes of patients.

I hope you now have a better appreciation for who you want on your All-Star Healthcare Team! If you start putting to use all (or at least some) of the tips I've recommended so far, you just might avoid having to contact some of these individuals. The important point is that you can and should assemble a top-notch team of medical professionals to advocate for your best health, in order for you to live your best, healthiest, and most productive life.

You may have been surprised to see a physical therapist high up on that list. I'll explain why in the next chapter.

CHAPTER 8

WHY GET PHYSICAL THERAPY FIRST?

Over the course of my 30+ years as a physical therapist (PT), the profession has grown tremendously. We've gone from bachelor-level programs to a doctoral-level program, so now to become a physical therapist, you must go through seven years of schooling to become an expert in the field of rehabilitation.

The body is meant to heal itself, and through exercise and education, you can get it better. The body is not meant to be cut open, nor is it meant to be given prescription drugs to solve every problem.

One of the main reasons for writing this book was to change the way most people think about physical therapy. Pain can be miserable. But it's even worse when it keeps you from doing the things you need, want, or love to do.

You should treat the causes of your pain and limitations, not just the symptoms. Pain is never due to a deficiency in painkillers, anti-inflammatories, or muscle relaxers. While those things have their place at times, they are generally just Band-Aids, and are not getting at the root cause of what is holding you back.

The client should also decide, along with their physical therapist (and not some administrator in a health insurance office), what type of treatment they receive. Great care makes no assumptions ever and meets people where they are. Physical therapy should be provided by an actual physical therapist, not just a physical therapy assistant, aide, or technician. And when you come in for an appointment, you should get far more than just 10 to 15 minutes of one-on-one time with them. The physical therapy experience should go way beyond the hands-on techniques we use, or the results you get.

Why It's a Good Idea to See a Physical Therapist for a Checkup

Healthcare consumers nowadays are becoming much smarter and more selective when it comes to spending their dollars. Many of my patients ask: "When should I call you?" My general answer is "Whenever you experience discomfort that doesn't quite seem right." Now I'm not talking about general muscle soreness after a workout, or after doing an activity you haven't done in a while. I'm talking about biking for 10 miles but feeling like you rode for 100 miles or jogging for 3 miles but feeling like you just ran a marathon.

I like to use the analogy of your car's Check Engine light. Pain is the brain's way of telling you that something isn't right, just as your car's Check Engine light tells you there's an issue with your car. Oftentimes, it is a simple problem, like you didn't tighten your gas cap. It could also be a serious issue, like the transmission. Regardless, the Check Engine light is simply a signal that something is not right, so you can seek out a professional mechanic to check out the problem.

Your body works in a similar fashion. Pain is the body's Check Engine light, a signal that something is not functioning properly. Take lower back pain, for example. A number of issues could be at play here—a herniated disc, a worsening spine condition such as degenerative disc disease, arthritis, or stenosis, or a sacroiliac (SI)/pelvic issue. Or the pain could be due to weakness in your glutes (butt muscles) when you swing a golf club.

Pain in the shoulder could be from a rotator cuff tear, impingement, or joint issue. Or it could simply be due to weakness in the shoulder blade muscles or rotator cuff, so they are not supporting your shoulder blade during overhead activities such as tennis and swimming.

Regardless, the important point is that the area of perceived pain is not always the source of the problem. Pain is a liar. So, it is extremely important that you see your body's "mechanic"—in this case, a physical therapist—to diagnose the problem and its source.

Remember, physical therapists are the experts in the musculoskeletal system; we are the functional movement experts of the body. We will watch you move, see how you perform specific tasks, and perform a thorough functional assessment to determine the root cause of your pain—and help you resolve it.

After all, you would not want your mechanic to simply reset your Check Engine light and send you home, which is basically what medication does. If you treat only your symptoms and not the source of the problem, your Check Engine light will come right back on when you resume normal activities.

Let's suppose you are one of the 25% of Americans who will suffer from low-back pain during any given 3-month period. After all, low-back pain is one of the most common reasons people visit a physician. While the majority of low-back pain episodes resolve on their own within 2 to 4 weeks, 25% of individuals will experience recurrent episodes within one year, often leading to the prevalence of chronic low-back pain, leading to a decrease in function and quality of life.

Let's take a look at what happens if you see your family physician first. In most cases, they will recommend imaging, meaning an X-ray or an MRI (magnetic resonance imaging). The problem is that the majority of Americans today over the age of 35 have bulging or herniated discs according to MRI results, yet these people are not symptomatic! This means that what you see on an X-ray or MRI image may not be the source of your pain. If your diagnostic test comes back positive, opioids are often prescribed for pain. When the opioids are no longer effective (and they quite often become habit-forming), you may be sent for painful spinal injections. And, you may be told that surgery is your only option.

Imagine that instead, you went to see your physical therapist first, rather than going to your physician. First off, physical therapists are trained to look for red flags, which may then lead them to recommend a particular diagnostic imaging test. But X-rays, CT scans, and MRIs are often not needed (and they don't always give us the whole picture). Starting physical therapy early will provide you with an active management approach that is based on movement. This is in direct opposition to the physician who prescribes opioids, which can foster a sense of dependency.

Going to a physical therapist first will also lower your overall healthcare costs. In a 2015 study, researchers found that individuals who were initially prescribed diagnostic imaging tests (such as X-rays and MRIs) for management of low-back pain instead of physical therapy ultimately paid more money. These same people were more likely to have injections, surgery, or visits to an emergency room, as compared to those who were first sent to physical therapists. In the year following their initial complaint to their physicians, the sample who started with physical therapy first spent an average of $1,871, compared to $6,664 for those who were first sent for an MRI. While there is a time and a place for diagnostic imaging, for most people, it is not in the early stages of care.

How to Make the Most of Your Physical Therapy Dollars

Insurance and government health programs can be expensive and frustrating for both consumers and providers. By far, the most common question I am asked first is "Do you take my insurance?" But what you should really be asking yourself is not "Will my insurance cover this?" but "Who can I trust to give me the best care for my money?"

A private-pay physical therapy practice is a far superior investment than an insurance-based physical therapy practice, even for clients who have health insurance. Contractual requirements from insurance-based health plans have intruded into the medical provider–client relationship. And the Affordable Care Act, with its more than 2,300 pages of regulations, has added even more layers of red tape, creating a bigger wedge between physical therapists and clients. Clients experience this wedge when they have to fill out more forms and provide more personal information. They feel it when sitting in waiting rooms much longer than they do in front of a physician. They experience less time with the primary care providers before they are passed on to support personnel. They know they are paying more but getting much less in terms of care.

Let's go over the major benefits to seeing a private-pay physical therapist.

Cost-effective care: Physical therapists have the extensive education and training to be your primary musculoskeletal and neuromuscular healthcare experts. For most individuals who experience movement difficulties, physical therapists are the providers of choice. Almost half of all Americans will experience some type of musculoskeletal episode each year. Skilled private-pay physical therapists are a third-party-free alternative for exceptional care and value.

Accessibility: All states now have some form of direct access, meaning you can bypass your physician or other healthcare provider to see a musculoskeletal or neuromuscular specialist (that is, a physical therapist) first, whereas many insurance companies require you to first see a physician or other healthcare professional who may not have the knowledge and expertise physical therapists have when dealing with movement issues. More often than not, the sooner a client can be evaluated and treated, the better the overall outcome.

Transparent, affordable pricing: For the self-pay client, finding a physical therapist who offers fair, simple, and transparent prices is crucial. Private-pay pricing eliminates the administrative costs for submitting claims to insurance companies. No more "We'll send the bill to your insurance company and see what they pay, then you will be responsible for the difference." Both parties will know the exact charges before any service takes place.

Protected client–physical therapist relationship: Imagine a physical therapy practice that does not demand your insurance card and photo ID before they even say hello. Or a practice where money does not get in the way of clients getting to know their physical therapist. Taking insurance middlemen out of the equation allows physical therapists to present themselves as empathetic professionals who understand the true cost of healthcare.

All clients are welcome: This includes everyone—insured or uninsured. Payment is by cash, check, or credit card. Clients are never rejected because of their insurance providers. In this type of setting, the true individual needs of each client can be met without outside interference.

Potential Risks of Not Seeing a Private-Pay Physical Therapist

Many individuals are currently seeking and receiving care and are paying out of pocket. Yet these people are not being seen by private-pay physical therapists. These individuals are seeking out massage therapists, chiropractors, acupuncturists, and other alternative healers—sometimes with alarming frequency and sometimes for issues that actually require medical intervention.

Unfortunately, many of these clients are seeking help from outside the system because they have become suspicious of mainstream medicine. They suspect that mainstream healthcare is all about the almighty dollar, and that physicians are puppets for the large pharmaceutical companies. They are tired of long waiting lists and brief encounters with doctors, physician assistants, nurse practitioners, and even insurance-based physical therapists.

But maybe more importantly, they feel unheard, disregarded, and shuttled from one specialist to the next, often assuming it is all in an effort to line the pockets of "the system."

They have given up on a system with fragmented care, where no one seems to want to take them on with the level of commitment they know they need and are actively seeking.

But herein lies the potential risks. Unfortunately, clients frequently fall into lengthy (often lifelong) passive treatment regimens, which over time can cost thousands of dollars. They begin to elevate their practitioners' opinions above sound evidence and clinical practice guidelines. There are horror stories about clients who continued to receive months and months of care from "alternative" healers, while all the while their cancer was spreading but very likely would have been identified as suspicious if only they had been seen by someone with the background to identify red flags.

This is where an exceptional private-pay physical therapist comes in. If only these individuals could receive first-class, evidence-based physical therapy delivered with empathy and a commitment to fostering self-care and empowerment—that would truly be the winning formula so many are desperately seeking.

As a private-pay physical therapist, my commitment is to maintain relationships with other medical professionals and refer to them when needed, whether it means recommending a diagnostic test to rule out pathology we suspect based on our skilled differential diagnoses or referring to an orthopaedic surgeon (or neurosurgeon) if our findings indicate the issue will most likely require surgical intervention. Thus, by delivering sound, evidence-based diagnoses and treatment, private-pay physical therapists most often provide the absolute best option for entering into the healthcare system.

Seven Signs You Need to Find a New Physical Therapist

If you've been through physical therapy, are currently going through it, or are looking to start a physical therapy regimen, pay close attention! Do you feel disappointed, dissatisfied, or frustrated with how you have been (or are being) treated by your physical therapist? Are you unhappy with the results you are (or are not) getting? If you answered yes to either or both of those questions, this next section will be extremely important to assist you in making a better decision about your health and, ultimately, getting back to the things you love.

When individuals are not treated well by their physical therapists or don't get desired results, they tend to write off physical therapy altogether, saying, "Physical therapy does not work for me, for my particular problem." This could possibly lead you (and your physician) to believe that medications, injections, and/or surgery are the answers, and that's not necessarily true.

Not all physical therapists are the same and, more often than not, physical therapy is the answer to your problem—provided you find the right physical therapist. Say you went to the blood bank to donate, and the phlebotomist stuck you with a needle but could not quite find your vein. So, they stuck you again and maybe even a third time!

Would you ever go back to that same phlebotomist again to have your blood drawn? I wouldn't! Would you think, "I don't believe donating blood is a positive experience, so I'm never doing that again!" I would hope not! It's not the blood donation that's the issue, it's the individual providing the service. It's the same exact notion with physical therapy—it's not that physical therapy is not right for you—it's just that you may need someone more proficient in using evidence-based research for healing your particular problem(s).

Now don't go beating yourself up over the fact that you may have chosen the wrong physical therapist. After all, people have no idea what the differences are between a good and bad physical therapist. Actually, many individuals don't have a clue when it comes to what a physical therapist actually does! I'm trying to get you to figure out if you do, in fact, need to change physical therapy providers to get you on the right track to recovery.

Here are my seven warning signs for determining whether you need to switch to a new physical therapist.

1.   *You are treated as a number on the schedule rather than a human being.*

   If you are one of four or five clients in the clinic being seen by the same physical therapist at the same time, you may feel like you are just being processed through "the system." Also, when you called to set up your first appointment, if the first 10 questions asked were about your insurance instead of your current problem, you may start to question whether they are truly interested in you as a person rather than a time slot on their schedule! One of the core values I practice is "People first, patients second."

2.   *You receive the same treatment every session.*

   The majority of clients should see improvement within the first two or three sessions. However, there are those clients who see absolutely no change after two or three sessions, yet the physical therapist will continue to perform the exact same treatment repeatedly. (Remember the definition of insanity— doing the same thing over and over but expecting different results.) Your physical therapist should alter and/or advance your treatments as you progress (or don't progress). Not doing so is a gross injustice!

3.   *You do not see progress.*

This piggybacks on #2. This should be fairly obvious, yet many clients continue to see their physical therapists without seeing significant progress. And this is not solely for making progress in eliminating your pain, but also in making progress toward attaining your goal(s), meaning what you want to accomplish as a result of physical therapy. Keep in mind that the first two or three sessions are often spent trying to reduce your pain to a manageable level so that the next several visits can focus more on your underlying problem(s).

4.   *You feel your true concerns and goals are not your own, and that you are not being heard.*

This relates to #1, but certainly needs its own listing. After all, isn't this the real reason you chose physical therapy in the first place, to get back to doing the things you love and enjoy? Unfortunately, this problem is not unique to physical therapy. How many times have you sat in a waiting room 10 times longer than you spent with your doctor?

When your physical therapist does not take the time to actively listen to your problems and concerns, they end up basing their treatment on what they think you need instead of what you actually need. The most effective treatment plans (and outcomes) occur when you and your physical therapist are on the same page in working toward your desired outcomes.

5. *There is no plan to get you back to doing what you love and want to do.*

In many instances, the primary objective of the physical therapist is to get you out of pain. But that is certainly not the true essence of physical therapy. As I say to my clients, "If all you're looking for is pain relief, take a pill. But if you're looking to get to the root (underlying) cause of your problem and eliminate it so it never comes back again, that's where I can help you."

6. *The majority of your treatment time is taken up by passive treatments.*

What do I mean by passive treatments? This is basically when you are sitting and not participating in your rehab program. You may be on a hot pack or an ice pack or be receiving electrical stimulation or mechanical traction. If the bulk of time you spend in the clinic is spent receiving passive treatments, there are much more cost-effective and time-effective treatment options to resolve your problem(s).

See if this sounds familiar. You are brought back for your treatment session and placed on a heating pad for 15–20 minutes. Then you receive a 5-minute ultrasound followed by a 5–10-minute general massage. You then perform your exercises (which you could do at home), maybe ride a bike or walk on a treadmill for 15–20 minutes, and maybe get ice and electrical stimulation at the end for 15 minutes.

If this is what you are experiencing (or have experienced), please know that this type of physical therapy will **NOT** give you the natural, long-term relief you are seeking. Unless the majority of your treatment program is hands-on manual therapy, then you aren't receiving the care you deserve.

7. *The majority of your treatment is spent with support staff.*

Here's the million-dollar question you need to ask yourself: "What are they doing for me in physical therapy that I can't do on my own at home?" If your response is something like "I'm really not sure" then you need to make a change. Not only are you wasting your time, but your money as well.

If you are going to an insurance-based provider and are responsible for a co-pay (which nowadays can be $50, $75, or even $100 per visit), you are paying the same amount whether you see the physical therapist for 10 minutes or 60. And if you're only seeing the physical therapist for 10 to 15 minutes, and your treatment lasts upwards of 1 hour, then you are spending three quarters of your time with support staff—a tech or an aide (in other words, an unlicensed professional). Wouldn't you prefer to spend 60 full minutes with the physical therapist without interruptions from other clients?

There are many good, qualified physical therapists who are willing and able to spend the quality time with you that you deserve. Know what to look for if you find yourself in the type of physical therapy clinic described in this section.

CHAPTER 9

DELAYING HEALTHCARE CHOICES CAN BE COSTLY AND PAINFUL

I spoke with a client not too long ago about choice—whether or not he should get a knee replacement. Now I certainly understand that some people just don't want to have to think about making such a major decision (even though they may be in tremendous discomfort and severely limited in what they can do, not to mention the limitations on where they can go). So, this gentleman (who was only in his mid-50s) saw his orthopaedic surgeon, who told him that he was actually in need of *both* knees needing to be replaced. (He was having discomfort in both knees, but clearly one was worse.) Mind you, the surgeon did not tell his patient to have the surgery—he was given plenty of time to think about it.

And think about it he did…for almost two years! Given the choice by his doctor, he stalled over making any decision. He finally did end up having both knees replaced two years later, the second knee three months after the first. (Nowadays, they often do bilateral knee replacements, avoiding the need to start over again from square one with rehab.) So, all was good after all, right? Well, not so fast!

During that two-year period of not making a decision to go ahead with the surgery that was clearly needed, this gentleman hobbled around, which led to lower back issues. Just three months after the second knee replacement, he suffered a collapsed vertebra, which not only caused excruciating back pain but sciatica (pain running down the back of the leg) as well. What happened next? Surgery to repair the collapsed vertebra. Which led to another four months of recovery from that surgery. Could things possibly have gotten any worse?

Unfortunately, yes! While walking in his yard, he stepped in a divot, causing a fracture in one of his foot bones. More surgery? Thankfully not this time. But he was placed in a walking boot for six weeks and had to use a walker, which likely aggravated his lower back further. (Not to mention the fact that his activity level was severely curtailed, leading to increased weakness in his back and legs.) Now I have to wonder—could all of this have been avoided?

Well, maybe and maybe not! What I can say is that our bodies are hardwired to move. Human movement is described through the concept of the kinetic chain. You most likely heard this concept as a child if you sang the song "the hip bone's connected to the leg bone, the leg bone's connected to the knee bone…" This kinetic chain concept states that each joint (or segment) of movement is affected by the joint (or segment) above and below. This is why in physical therapy the location of the pain is often not the source (or cause) of the problem. So quite possibly this gentleman could have started out with a hip problem, and it was his knees (the joint directly below them in the kinetic chain) that took the brunt of the forces.

All of these "abnormal" forces could have caused the problems in his knees, lower back, and foot. Now think about walking around like this for an additional two years while this gentleman did not make a decision about the best course of action. Of course, some of you out there might say he was just unlucky. Unfortunately, luck had nothing to do with his progression. This is really better explained as the "domino effect." I have seen it time and time again over my 30+ years as a physical therapist, where individuals procrastinate over important healthcare decisions.

My point here is not the fact that an individual's choice regarding their own healthcare should be made by someone else—absolutely not! But people would save a lot of time, money, and pain if they were given reliable information in order to make better, more educated, and more informed decisions about how their bodies really work! I truly do believe that most individuals want to have their health restored and activity levels maintained and do really want to go ahead with procedures such as joint replacements (especially for hips and knees). It's simply the fear of the unknown that they don't want to have to live with!

I hope you now have a better appreciation for not only what physical therapy is, but all of the problems and issues we address and resolve daily. Remember the two words that describe a physical therapist: movement specialist! This should help you to keep us top of mind if you have any questions about what I have covered.

Go back and look at the chapter topics: pain, exercise, nutrition, stress reduction and mental well-being, and rest and recovery. Now you know that physical therapists are your best choice to address all those areas!

Conclusion

It was truly a labor of love to write this book. All throughout my 30+ year career as a physical therapist, I've prided myself on educating my clients, in terms of both healing and prevention. Every one of you has a choice regarding your health. And with the constant changes and uncertainty in today's healthcare market, it is more important than ever to take an active role in your health.

Start being proactive about your healthcare instead of reactive, like way too many out there. Life is full of choices, and I hope this book gives the control back to you. After all, we're living longer and working longer, and have more healthcare responsibilities than ever before, both for ourselves and our loved ones.

By following the simple suggestions laid out in this book, my hope is to get you back to doing the things you want and love to do—back to being normal again! After all, you should do the things now that your future self will thank you for. Healing is not a moment but a lifelong process. And now you have the tools to live your best life!

About the Author

Dr. David A. Wilderman, PT, DPT, MS, founder of Wilderman Physical Therapy, was born and raised in Wilmington, Delaware. After graduating from the University of Delaware, he went on to earn a Master of Science in Physical Therapy from Arcadia University and a Doctor of Physical Therapy from Boston University.

Dr. Wilderman's professional experience includes several start-up clinics in Baltimore, MD, Shrewsbury, PA, and Wilmington, DE. He was a partner in Shrewsbury Physical Therapy from 2000–2008, then left to open Wilderman and Associates Physical Therapy, PC, in Shrewsbury, PA, in 2009. He sold the practice in late 2011 to return to his home state of Delaware.

Dr. Wilderman's specialties include:

- orthopaedic rehabilitation with a particular emphasis on neck, spine, and shoulder rehab
- sports medicine rehabilitation
- neurological rehabilitation
- chronic headache relief
- TMJ rehabilitation
- wellness and preventative programs

He has been an active member of the American Physical Therapy Association (APTA) since 1984, as well as the orthopaedic, sports, and private-practice sections of the APTA.

Dr. Wilderman founded Wilderman Physical Therapy in order to practice in a setting that embodies his philosophy of treatment. He believes in the use of education, individualized attention, and client input to help his clients alleviate their pain and physical impairments. Receiving physical therapy at Wilderman Physical Therapy enhances the potential results following an injury or surgery, providing improved function, minimized disability, and less time away from work and leisure activities.

When Wilderman Physical Therapy was created, there was one goal in mind: to provide the ultimate care to clients by giving them superior value in terms of service. When most people research products and services, they generally look at three factors: cost, quality, and convenience. Oftentimes, individuals will sacrifice at least one of these factors in their decisions. The problem is, the current trend in health insurance is toward higher co-pays and deductibles. As a result, many patients are paying out of pocket for the majority of their care but are not getting the best value for their dollars.

Many of my clients have had prior attempts at treatment, whether from physical therapy, chiropractic, pain management (including painful epidural injections), massage therapy, acupuncture, or family physicians treating their symptoms conservatively with medication. But they were not completely satisfied with the outcomes, and still not back to their prior functional levels.

So how am I different?

For starters, you will spend one full hour with me, a licensed Doctor of Physical Therapy. You will see no other support staff (or other patients, for that matter), nor will you perform repetitious exercises that you could do on your own at home. Your treatment will not be dictated by what your insurance company will or will not cover—this is one of the primary reasons I have chosen to be private-pay and not to accept insurance other than Medicare. I provide therapeutic outcomes that are in line with your goals to attain maximal success in getting you back to the activities you love. Bottom line—fewer visits (**cost**), higher standards of care (**quality**), and appointments only one or two times per week (**convenience**).

If you have further questions regarding anything covered in this book, I would love to hear from you. I can best be reached by email at drdave@wildermanpt.com. I welcome all feedback, comments, and questions, and will respond to each one personally. For more information, please go to my website at www.wildermanphysicaltherapy.com.